The Medical Triangle

The Medical Triangle

Physicians, Politicians,

and the Public

·

ELI GINZBERG

HARVARD UNIVERSITY PRESS
Cambridge, Massachusetts
London, England
1990

Library of Congress Cataloging-in-Publication Data

Ginzberg, Eli, 1911–
   The medical triangle: physicians, politicians, and the public /
Eli Ginzberg.
      p.   cm.
   Includes bibliographical references.
   ISBN 0-674-56325-5 (alk. paper)
   1. Medical policy—United States. 2. Medical care—United States.
I. Title.
   [DNLM: 1. Delivery of Health Care—United States. 2. Health Policy—
United States. 3. Health Services—economics—United States.
W 84 AA1 G4m]
RA418.3.U6G56 1990
362.1′0973—dc20
DNLM/DLC   89-24566
for Library of Congress   CIP

To
David E. Rogers
A Friend of Two Decades

Contents

IV · Patients' Needs and Resources

V · Health Agenda Issues

Preface

One way to assess the highly volatile health care scene is to focus on what is new and different and project small beginnings into major trends. With equal justification, one can stand back and question whether the many new departures and changes are really that important considering that the basic contours of our health care system have not been altered significantly. As the essays following (all of which represent work completed after 1985) indicate, I have taken a middle course, seeking to be sensitive to the new without becoming overimpressed with the longer-term implications of each innovation for restructuring the operations of our extant health care system. Admittedly, the cumulative effects of many new developments may at some point generate sufficient force to alter the foundations and the superstructure of our long-established and well-entrenched system. But the prospect for it to remain reasonably intact for some additional time to come is the more probable scenario, given the broad satisfaction of most, though surely not all, Americans with the quantity and quality of their health care services.

The tension between system maintenance and system change pervades all of the essays, and I have tried my best to focus on analysis, not ideology. This does not mean that I lack ideas on what ought to be changed if the health care delivery system were to become more effective, more efficient, and more equitable. But my principal intention has been to provide the reader with a broader and clearer understanding of the multiple forces that are jostling each other and the probabilities that attach to one or another's gaining dominance in the near and longer term.

Health care, broadly conceived, is a subsystem of a larger societal matrix involving in the first instance members of the medical profession who, alone by law, have the right to diagnose and treat patients. In this context politicians too are important players, since the three levels of government, with the federal government in the lead, account for 40 percent of the annual financing of the system, which in 1988 had a total cost of about $540 billion. And the public, with over 1 billion visits to physicians a year and with about 34 million hospital admissions, is clearly a key party.

Some analysts insist that one more major player must be identified: employers who provide health care benefits to their employees that cover roughly 30 percent of the annual health care bill. I see no reason to challenge the inclusion of employers, although it is worth pointing out that only in the last few years, really since the recession of the early 1980s, have employers sought to modify the system with the aim of controlling their costs, so far with small success.

The major themes in this book fall roughly into five groupings. In Part I—"The Changing Health Care System"—the reader is reminded that the core institutions of the U.S. health care system have been the community hospital and physicians who have long practiced in a fee-for-service mode. Both are currently under attack from a variety of forces and it is unlikely that the process of destabilization can be reversed. The open issue is how far and how fast it will proceed.

The exciting but short life of for-profit medicine is a powerful reminder that every new development in health care is not necessarily of lasting importance. But as the last three chapters in Part I make clear, it would be an equally egregious mistake to overlook the extent to which changes in medical technology, the expectations of the public, and the ability of politicians to respond are altering the health care system and are likely to alter it still more in the years ahead.

In Part II I focus on the academic health center, the lead institution of the U.S. health care system, which has been the principal home for innovation in medical research and medical care since the end of World War II and even earlier. The most important of these centers have annual budgets in the half-billion range with work forces that number in the multiple thousands. Their economic muscle is a precondition for their professional leadership, and in turn their professional accomplishments have strengthened their leadership role. But in a period in which new dollars for health care are harder to come by, their future vitality cannot be taken for granted.

The last three chapters in Part II review the notable weakening in the role of foundations as agents of change in the health care arena, a consequence primarily of their modest dollar inputs. Chapter 8 provides an evaluation of a carefully crafted foundation effort to improve the delivery of health care to inner-city poor people, the outcome of which was equivocal. And Chapter 9, focusing on New York City, traces and evaluates the impact of very large dollar increases (threefold in constant dollars) upon health care between 1965 and 1985 in terms of who benefited and how much. The answer turned out to be: everybody who had a place at the trough, from academic health centers to the housekeeping personnel in nursing homes, and patients who required more ambulatory, acute, or long-term care.

Part III deals with medical education, the physician supply, and nursing. It demonstrates in the first instance the modest role that analysis has played in determining future needs for physicians as against the role of "politics," meaning the changing attitudes and behavior of key groups that control medical school admissions. And Chapter 10 is a reminder of the traditionalism that has dominated medical education since the Flexner approach came to the fore in the second decade of this century. It is still in full control as the century nears its end. The nursing shortage that the nation was suffering at the close of the 1980s is a problem whose genesis and resolution are embedded in the context of the wider labor market opportunities for women, changing demographics, and the changing health care system, which define the critical issues that face the nurse leadership.

In Part IV five chapters deal sequentially with high-need patients for whom there is currently limited financing and, at best, only restricted opportunities for major changes in the future. But the thrust of the analysis is to suggest that more money alone would help only a little, not a lot, to resolve the serious problems facing patients with catastrophic illness, cancer, those suffering the infirmities of old age, the mentally ill, and those who are chronically poor.

Part V deals with some more or less intractable problems for which current and prospective health policy will be hard pressed to find and implement useful solutions. The three chapters examine the balancing of equity and efficiency in the provision of health care, the unsuccessful pursuit of cost containment (now in its third decade), and the lack of consensus among physicians, politicians, and the public about the major issues on the nation's health agenda. In the absence of such consensus, the existing system will continue to be pulled in a great many different directions by the key players to the growing dissatisfaction of all.

Acknowledgments

My long-term associate, Miriam Ostow, was coauthor of the published articles that have been reprinted in the book as Chapters 8 and 9. Moreover, she contributed to each of the articles out of which this book has been constructed. I want to acknowledge my deep and continuing appreciation for a collegial relationship of more than two decades.

Chapter 10, written with Robert Ebert, formed the centerpiece of a special supplement of *Health Affairs* in the spring of 1988. Dr. Ebert graciously agreed to my reprinting our joint essay as part of this volume.

The notes provide details as to where the several chapters first appeared and record the permissions received to republish them. All of the chapters except for 5 and 18 have been previously published, or are in the process of being published. They are reprinted here with a few minor stylistic or editorial changes.

During the years that these articles were being prepared and published, the Conservation of Human Resources Project, Columbia University, received liberal support from the Robert Wood Johnson Foundation and the Commonwealth Fund, assistance for which I am deeply grateful. This volume is a by-product of that support.

I profited often from the support of Anna Dutka. Sylvia Leef and Shoshana Vasheetz saw the successive versions through our reproduction system, for which I am much in their debt.

E. G.
August 1989

· I ·

The Changing
Health Care
System

The Destabilization of Health Care

During the last fifteen years there have been many signs of the increasing destabilization of the health care system in the United States. Between the Flexner report in 1910 and the 1970s, a period of six decades, the system had been characterized by a remarkable stability that reflected three factors: the dominance of the medical profession; local sponsorship of community hospitals; and the practice of cross-subsidization, which enabled physicians and hospitals to care for many of the poor by overcharging the affluent. The established system was able to adjust to new opportunities while protecting and fostering important societal values.

The flexibility of the system was demonstrated by the transformation of community hospitals from institutions of care to institutions of cure, the restructuring of the medical profession when general practitioners were replaced by specialists, and the proliferation of academic health centers heavily involved in biomedical research funded by liberal grants from the federal government. Even with the advantage of hindsight, it is not clearly understood how the established system accommodated these pervasive changes while maintaining its underlying structure and organization.

For the last twenty-five years, however, since shortly after the laws establishing Medicare and Medicaid were passed, the health care system has been increasingly buffeted and battered. A large and growing proportion of the medical profession now consists of physician employees of nonprofit hospitals or corporate enterprises, rather than private practitioners;[1] for-profit and nonprofit hospital chains threaten the role of many autonomous community hospitals; the broad risk pool that enabled persons in poor health to acquire health insurance at a reasonable cost is being increasingly segmented as more and more large employers move to self-insurance;[2] and cross-subsidization is evaporating in the face of intensified price competition, with adverse consequences for the poor and the near-poor.[3]

In the late 1960s the federal government took initial steps to control steeply rising health care expenditures. Since then, other payers joined the government and the effort has intensified. But in our frenetic pursuit of the elusive goal of cost containment, many important values in the established system have been lost or are at risk. Undermining the existing structure to accomplish cost control might be considered a reasonable trade-off. But to destabilize a functioning system of health care without achieving corresponding gains in controlling costs, as I believe to be the case,[4] is a dubious result.

The destabilization process was potentiated by forces unleashed by the Medicare-Medicaid reforms of the mid-1960s and by the policy changes implemented in recent years. But already in the pre-Medicare era latent forces were at work that would, over time, contribute to the unsettling of the status quo. The two most important were the rapid increases in the numbers of physicians in the training pipeline and the consequences of broader and deeper hospital and health insurance.

In the first decades after World War II, the states moved aggressively to establish new medical schools and to increase the number of graduates of existing schools. In the early 1960s the federal government, after years of providing indirect support to medical schools by means of grants from the National Institutes of Health, moved directly and vigorously to enlarge the supply of physicians.[5]

One of the principal constraints on the rate of change in the existing system—the tightness of the physician supply—was thus undermined, although it would take a few years before the consequences of the increasing supply of physicians would be felt. Among the obstacles to the growth of prepayment plans during the early postwar decades were the desirable options of young physicians in the fee-for-service sector. But the doubling of the supply of new physicians in the 1970s would eventually introduce changes in modes of practice.[6]

The second force that threatened the extant system was the rapid increase in health and hospital insurance characterized by "first-dollar" coverage. In 1971 Martin Feldstein called attention to the danger that broad insurance would result in overutilization, which would lead in turn to waste and cost inflation.[7] Some years later, Alain Enthoven explored this issue in depth and called attention to the federal tax subsidy for employers and employees that further reduced incentives to economize in buying health insurance and in using health care services.[8]

Each of these developments—a larger supply of physicians and improved insurance coverage—was likely to alter the health care system, but neither factor alone nor both together were sufficient to destabilize it.

The Medicare Era

The Medicare-Medicaid reforms and their direct and unanticipated consequences precipitated the process of destabilization. With regard to hospitals, third-party payments rose from 77 to 91 percent of total costs,[9] and this lessened the long-standing preoccupation of trustees and hospital administrators with financial matters. Moreover, the new strong cash flows, which promised to increase from year to year, enabled nonprofit hospitals to break away from the philanthropic sources that had in the past covered a large part of their capital outlays.[10] Large hospitals (and many smaller ones) were able to go to the tax-free bond market and, on the basis of their prospective reimbursements, borrow all the money they needed for expansion, improvements, and modernization.[11] The hospital sector was on easy street for the first time. One aspect of this situation that escaped notice, however, was the erosion of interest, power, and influence of many boards of trustees. Hospital administrators, acting largely alone, could meet the needs of their professional staffs for new and improved facilities, technology, and services. A major source of strength in the old system, a concerned and committed community leadership, had been weakened.[12]

The new affluence did not remain restricted to the predominant nonprofit sector for long. Shortly after the passage of Medicare and Medicaid, a new player entered the field—the for-profit hospital chain. Since the health care sector was awash in dollars, the well-managed new for-profit companies had little difficulty in finding attractive niches, primarily in the South and West, where most states followed a charge-reimbursement rather than a cost-reimbursement formula.[13] With the equity market looking favorably on their prospects, the growth companies were able to obtain additional capital that helped fuel their growth. Congress also lent a helping hand by permitting Medicare reimbursement to be based on values inflated by acquisitions and improvements. Congress also provided the for-profit hospital chains a generous return on their equity investment.[14]

In less than a decade, the for-profit hospital chains increased their ownership of acute-care beds from 55,000 (in 1976) to 111,000 (in 1984); by 1984 they were also managing another 41,000 beds.[15] Some informed observers have prophesied that before the end of the century the health care system would be dominated by some ten to twenty "megafirms."[16]

The Post-Medicare Era

During the 1970s and the first half of the 1980s, many forces old and new combined to help destabilize the health care system. The emergence and substantial growth of for-profit hospital chains weakened the hegemony of the community hospital in many parts of the country, and the emergence of potential surpluses of both physicians and hospitals resulted in corresponding threats to the continued dominance of these two key power centers. The establishment of professional standards review organizations (PSROs) and certificate of need (CON) legislation in the early 1970s,[17] together with the failed attempts of the Carter administration to place a ceiling on annual capital outlays for hospitals, were early warning signs of a more aggressive role of the federal government. When Medicare was first enacted, President Lyndon Johnson had assured the American Medical Association that the federal government would not unsettle the established system by interfering with the traditional patient-physician relationship. The fact that President Richard Nixon took the lead as early as 1971 to obtain congressional support for the expansion of health maintenance organizations shows how quickly Johnson's promise was broken.

The 1970s ended with the established system still very much in place, although the signs pointed to a weakening of its foundations. When President Ronald Reagan took office in 1981, the new administration announced that it would rely on the competitive market rather than on federal regulation to shape the nation's health care system.[18] Furthermore, it gave notice that it would seek early congressional support for a radical cutback in federal expenditures for health care. However, the administration secured congressional approval for only some of its cuts, and it never introduced a broad, strategic proposal for reform based on competition.

Nonetheless, competitive forces came to play a much larger part, principally because of the following factors: the rapid growth of entrepreneurial activities by both for-profit and nonprofit health care organizations, primarily in ambulatory care facilities; the explosive growth of health maintenance organizations, preferred-provider organizations, and other forms of managed care; and the determined and largely successful efforts of the business sector to renegotiate its health benefit plans and, in the process, to provide incentives for its employees to enroll in alternatives to fee-for-service arrangements. Moreover, a growing proportion of large corporations moved to self-insurance.

It would be difficult to find another two-year period comparable to 1981–1983 with respect to the number of innovations in health care financing and delivery. But two more events must be noted because they contributed substantially to the processes of destabilization: the institution of prospective payment for the hospitalization of Medicare beneficiaries and the growing excess of the two critical resources—physicians and hospital beds.

The cumulative interaction of these multiple trends and forces substantially destabilized the three foundation blocks of the established system—the nonprofit community hospital; the dominance of the physician in therapeutic decision-making; and cross-subsidization, which had previously enabled many providers to care for substantial numbers of poor patients. Many community hospitals, faced with a rapidly declining patient census, joined one of the large chains, which soon claimed to have a membership encompassing one third of all nonprofit hospitals.

Other hospitals organized for-profit affiliates to help them keep afloat in a shrinking market for inpatient care, and still others merged or changed their missions.[19]

Many new doctors found themselves confronting a market that was much more competitive than they had expected. In the face of steeply rising malpractice premiums and the dearth of opportunities for starting a practice, many recently certified physicians settled for salaried employment, often with a corporate enterprise that paid them $35,000 to $40,000 a year.[20] Almost all physicians were affected by the rules of the newly organized peer-review organizations and the guidelines for treatment that the hospitals in which they practiced promulgated in response to the system of payment based on diagnosis-related groups. Physicians also faced a difficult choice in 1983, when they had to decide whether to accept a Medicare fee freeze or risk later a delay in the adjustment of their fee profile.

The combination of corporate self-insurance, the tightening of insurers' payment practices, and the growth of volume discounting by preferred-provider organizations reduced the revenues that earlier had enabled many providers to cross-subsidize the health care of the poor. Many hospitals thus became more inclined to "dump" patients with limited or no insurance in public hospitals, a practice which recent federal and state legislation has sought to control. The antidumping legislation relating to seriously ill patients that was recently passed by selected states and the federal government reflects the difficulties many hospitals encounter when confronted by patients without insurance coverage.

The Dialectics of Destabilization

One remaining question is whether the accelerating forces for destabilization are likely to continue unchecked until most of the earlier system of health care fades into history, or whether such forces will be slowed down, arrested, even reversed. It has been difficult to discern the constants within the confusions of the recent past, and even more difficult to discern the thrust of the present, which will set the directions and limitations for the future.

In the case of the nonprofit community hospitals, we can

probably anticipate the disappearance of many small hospitals and the resizing of the total hospital plant. I do not expect, however, that the continued growth of the for-profit hospital chains will have a serious effect on the future of the community hospitals. These chains have not enlarged their proportion of acute care beds since 1980 and are not likely to do so in the future, since studies indicate that they do not operate more effectively or efficiently than nonprofit hospitals.[21] Moreover, there are signs that the trustees of many community hospitals are paying closer attention to their institutions' present and future roles. In addition, many broad-based business coalitions may be the harbingers of greater community commitment. It is surely premature to contemplate the swift demise of the community hospital.

The forces affecting the medical profession are more difficult to assess. Clearly, the earlier untrammeled freedom of the profession to determine how, where, and for how long patients would be treated is being circumscribed by new rules, regulations, and protocols. But it is too early to conclude that all "interferences" are necessarily bad for physicians or patients, even as they may save payers money.

On the other hand, several new factors—including the ever increasing number of physicians entering the profession, the decreased opportunities for residents to practice their specialties, the unchecked rise in malpractice-insurance premiums, the standardization of medical practice in prepayment and managed care systems, the marketing tactics pursued by for-profit medical enterprises, and the financial stake of physicians through ownership or partnership in facilities and equipment to which they refer their patients—suggest that the environment and the ethics of medical care are changing and will continue to change. During this time of destabilization, there is a risk that important values may be lost; this will depend on the quality of the medical leadership and the response of the public.

Another serious concern is that the care of the poor can no longer be financed as broadly as in the past through cross-subsidization. It should be noted that after the cutbacks of 1981–1983, many states extended and improved their Medicaid coverage. A considerable number of states have also established all-payer pools out of which they reimburse hospitals that provide care to disproportionately large numbers of poor patients. The secretary of the Department of Health and Human Services (HHS) is under a congressional directive to revise the payment schedule for Medicare to reflect the "disproportionate share" of charity care provided by selected hospitals.[22]

The foregoing review raises hard questions that require at least tentative answers. Will the forces encouraging further destabilization overwhelm the points of resistance that have begun to emerge? Why would it be bad if destabilization continued? What are the important values embedded in the inherited health care system that we should continue to protect?

In regard to the first question, it is difficult to estimate how large a segment of the middle class will join a managed-care system, even if it is a little less expensive than fee for service. My own guess is that the managed-care system will continue to grow although not at a precipitous rate, and that it may level off in the range of 25–33 percent. If this guess proves to be correct, the forces for destabilization will begin to abate.

But suppose my estimate is too low, and managed care comes to dominate the system. What would be so bad about trying to control costs, prevent unnecessary hospitalizations, and shorten hospital stays, insisting that physicians use reasonable (not excessive) amounts of resources, and making still other departures from the good old days, which surely constituted no utopia?

There would be little wrong with these departures if they represented the whole story. But if further destabilization resulted in a proliferation of corporate practices of medicine in which most physicians become employees, in a system in which protocol medicine was the norm, in an erosion of local voluntarism in hospital care, and in the elimination of cross-subsidization, creating additional obstacles to access for the poor, then a great deal would be lost.

My greatest concern is that we have been pursuing contradictory policies that are adding to our problems. The competitive market is an opponent, not an ally, of cost containment.[23] When capacity, advertising, and marketing increase, the boundaries of the system are expanded, duplication of costly services is encouraged, and the public is pushed to consume more health care services than it needs. Companies that are self-insured and that press for experience-rated premiums make it more difficult to bring poor patients into the system and to keep them there. Neither competition nor cost containment will ensure the maintenance of medical research and medical education, on which further advances in therapeutics depend.[24] Continued destabilization must be slowed and then reversed if we are not to undermine what has proved to be a highly satisfactory and effective system of care for most Americans.

· 2 ·

For-Profit Medicine

On the organizational side, the past two decades have been a period of emergence and growth of for-profit health care delivery corporations, initially in hospitals and later extending to the provision of ambulatory care services. But only a few years after the advocates of the new corporations prophesied that the nation's health care system would soon be dominated by a few "SuperMeds,"[1] the four largest for-profit hospital chains—Hospital Corporation of America, National Medical Enterprises, Humana, and American Medical International—began scaling down their operations and spinning off substantial segments.[2]

What forces led to the growth of these new health care delivery companies and their high profits? What assumptions were made about their productivity and profitability that time proved false? With the advantage of lengthened perspective, what is the prognosis for for-profit medicine?

Setting the Boundaries

For-profit enterprises have always operated in the health care arena. Starting with the manufacture and marketing of drugs and medical equipment and appliances, they later invaded medical education. In 1910 the Flexner report found that 28 of the more than 150 medical schools in the United States were stock companies, operated by entrepreneurs who were primarily concerned with making money. Another 50 were independent institutions not related to universities, most of them controlled by practitioners who sought to capture the tuition income for themselves. In his recommendation to eliminate substandard schools by bringing medical education under the control of state boards, Flexner stated: "Medicine, curative and preventive, has indeed no analogy with business. Like the Army, the police, or the social worker, the medical profession is supported for a benign, not a selfish, for a protective, not an exploiting, purpose."[3]

Between the Flexner report and the passage of the legislation establishing Medicare and Medicaid, a period of fifty-five years, for-profit medical enterprises engaged primarily in the manufacture and sale of drugs, medical equipment, and appliances and in selling health insurance policies to employers and individual persons. In 1965, these activities accounted for $8.1 billion out of a total national health expenditure of $41.9 billion, or just over 19 percent.[4]

There was also a modest for-profit presence in the areas of acute hospital care, psychiatric hospitals, and nursing homes. In terms of nongovernmental acute care capacity, nonprofit hospitals accounted for 515,000 beds and for-profit hospitals for 47,000—a ratio of roughly 11:1.[5] Including its hospital activities, the total share of national expenditures on health of the for-profit sector came to 22 percent in 1965. Government accounted for 26 percent, and the remaining 52 percent represented the mainstream—the earnings of fee-for-service professionals, primarily physicians and dentists (30 percent), and combined expenditures of nonprofit hospitals, nursing homes, and the marketing and administrative outlays of the nonprofit Blue Cross and Blue Shield organizations (22 percent).[6] Clearly, in the direct delivery of health care services to the American people, the for-profits had never been more than minor players. Nonprofit hospitals and fee-for-service professionals dominated the U.S. health care system.

The shortage of hospital beds, particularly in areas of the country that had large population increases, together with the introduction of Medicare and Medicaid (which turned most of those admitted to hospitals into paying patients) created the establishment and growth of the for-profit hospital chains. In the decade after the passage of the legislation establishing Medicare and Medicaid, the number of nonprofit acute care hospital beds increased from 515,000 to 659,000, or by 28 percent. During the same decade the for-profit hospital sector grew from 47,000 to 73,000 beds (55 percent).[7]

The for-profit chains bought or constructed hospitals in states with favorable reimbursement environments, where insurers tended to reimburse on the basis of charges or at least on the basis of costs. In 1985, 60.7 percent of the acute care beds of the for-profit chains were located in just five states: California, Florida, Louisiana, Tennessee, and Texas.[8] The for-profit hospitals tended to be located in affluent suburbs, where the pressure to provide charity care was reduced, and in general they avoided high-cost, low-profit services such as outpatient departments and emergency rooms or teaching programs.

The expansion of the for-profit chains was further stimulated by congressional authorization of the inclusion of a return on equity in reimbursement for care provided to Medicare beneficiaries. Medicare also provided for interest payments and higher depreciation rates on properties previously purchased by the for-profit chains.[9]

Increasing demand for hospital care, along with third-party payments that covered 90 percent of all in-patient expenditures (which made a hospital virtually a risk-free enterprise) and favorable reimbursement arrangements with private insurers, Blue Cross, state agencies, and Medicare (for operating as well as capital expenses) created and sustained strong cash flows. Nevertheless, the rapid expansion of the for-profit chains could not have been achieved solely, or even largely, through retained earnings. The hospital chains needed—and obtained—entry to the equity market. With strong assistance from the investment banking community, which is always on the lookout for promising initiatives, Wall Street looked favorably on the for-profit hospital chains, and for a number of years the results justified its enthusiasm.

The answer to what caused the initial rapid growth and high profits of the for-profit companies can be found in their strong entrepreneurial response to the expanding demand for hospital care, funded by Medicare and Medicaid and broadened and deepened by private insurance. This environment provided the newcomers with the opportunity to find niches in states with favorable reimbursement policies. Their progress was further fueled by the receptiveness of the stock market, which gave them access to large amounts of equity capital.

Basic Assumptions

It was not easy for the for-profit hospital chains to legitimize their role in health care delivery, and they were careful to deal with physicians as independent professionals, impinging little or not at all on their freedom to make decisions. As the for-profits developed a strong track record of rapid growth, high profits, and substantial appreciation in the value of their stocks, they, their friends on Wall Street, and increasing numbers of health care analysts sought to explain their remarkable performance.

First and foremost, it was thought that for-profit hospital chains were able to exploit economies of scale, not only through their ownership of several hospitals but also through the additional volume of care they provided in the hospitals that they managed under contract. Clearly, scale has advantages—for instance, in the purchasing of supplies and equipment, in the development and execution of building plans, and in the control of inventories.

A second explanation emphasized the ability of for-profit chains to put in place a strong management structure and to reap the benefits that it provided. A rapidly expanding, profitable hospital chain was in a better position to attract, train, promote, and retain capable hospital administrators than an unaffiliated community hospital experiencing modest growth.

A closely related but still distinguishable point was what analysts perceived as the greater ability of a profitable hospital chain to develop and install strong planning and control systems. These systems were supported by computer hardware and software capable of providing the data that were essential for improved decision making.

Fourth, with labor costs accounting for more than half of all hospital expenditures, for-profit hospitals were able to introduce tighter controls on the use of nursing and support staff and to develop company-wide policies aimed at improved use of personnel. This assumption, too, had some basis in theory and in fact. Administrators, chief nurses, and computer experts who proved themselves at a small hospital often had the opportunity to move to a larger institution where they could be more productive.

Finally, for-profit hospitals, free of the traditions, regulations, and inertia characteristic of their competitors in the nonprofit sector, could respond more quickly and effectively to the expressed and latent demands of patients for a more pleasant, more supportive environment that offered more attractive accommodations, better food, liberalized visiting hours, and other amenities.

These five factors should have led to lower costs, lower prices, and a growth in market share for the for-profit chains. However, the chains never succeeded in gaining a competitive cost advantage over the nonprofit hospitals, and they pursued a pricing policy that was geared to optimizing their profits. They relied on acquisitions to gain market share.[10]

The for-profit hospital chains were managed by businessmen whose entrepreneurial expertise was in real estate, construction, and financing; they had to learn how to run hospitals through trial and error. The fact that hospital care is a local service with labor accounting for between 50 and 60 percent of total costs seriously limited the potential gains from economies of scale. Removing a patient's appendix is inherently different from manufacturing an automobile or franchising Kentucky Fried Chicken. Moreover, the for-profit chains did not escape the propensity of most large corporations to accumulate excessive staff, a tendency that raised expenses more than it provided added value.[11]

The for-profit chains did well in the 1970s by virtue of the strong cash flows that underpinned their rapid growth. The 1980s brought a softening in the demand for in-patient care, a shift to ambulatory care, and a tightening of reimbursement policies. Between 1975 and 1980 admissions to acute care hospitals increased from 33.4 million to 36.1 million (8 percent), and days of care rose from 257.5 million to 274.7 million (6.7 percent). In the succeeding five years, from 1980 to 1985, admissions dropped from 36.1 to 33.4 million (7.5 percent), and total days of care from 274.7 to 237.5 million (13.5 percent).[12]

The for-profit chains were lifted and lowered by the changing tide. Between 1975 and 1980, their admissions increased by 19.6

percent and their total days of care by 17.8 percent. In the five years from 1980 to 1985, they experienced an increase of 2.5 percent in admissions but a 3.8 percentage decline in days of care. Their rates of occupancy dropped sharply, from 65.2 percent in 1980 to 52.1 percent in 1985 (a decline of 20 percent).[13]

Starting in 1981, when the federal government allowed the states greater leeway in setting rates for their Medicaid beneficiaries, the reimbursement environment became less favorable. At about the same time, employers began to rewrite their health benefit plans, mandating deductibles and coinsurance so that their employees would share some of the costs of hospital care. Many employers also introduced utilization review, with the aim of moderating the steep increases in their hospital expenditures. In 1983 the diagnosis-related groups (DRGs) were adopted, and Congress reduced by one third the return on equity that for-profit hospitals were permitted to earn, as a preliminary to eliminating this factor entirely in 1990. The decline in demand for inpatient care and the tightening of reimbursement policies signaled trouble ahead in the hospital environment. The for-profit chains suddenly found themselves handicapped in a number of ways.

They had for the most part failed to attract to their staffs the best-established and most prestigious members of the medical profession, who played the key role in determining where patients were admitted. Nor had their boards attracted the community business leaders who could intervene with local or state government officials when intervention was necessary or desirable. Furthermore, the fact that most for-profit hospitals lacked graduate training programs meant that they were less well positioned to attract patients requiring tertiary care or Medicaid patients whose care was largely in the hands of residents. Many of the competitive weaknesses of the for-profit hospital chains had been obscured during the upbeat 1970s, but they came to the fore in the less favorable 1980s.

As for capital funding, the apparent advantages of the for-profit chains over the nonprofit hospitals, predicated on their ability to tap the private financial markets, had narrowed as the nonprofits gained more access to the bond market; the contribution of bonds to capital needs of nonprofit hospitals rose from 30 percent in the 1960s and 1970s to 60 percent in the 1980s.[14]

Finally, the nonprofit hospitals saw advantages to adopting some of the organizational and management practices of the for-profit sector, from establishing chain operations to instituting new information systems.

The Future of the For-Profit Sector

The logic of rapid growth led the for-profit chains to move beyond the acquisition and construction of acute care hospitals. Some established a presence overseas;[15] others contracted to buy or manage academic health centers;[16] still others moved aggressively to specialize, acquiring psychiatric hospitals, rehabilitation facilities, and addiction-treatment centers that were expected from the DRG regulations in 1983 and that continue, at least for the present, to generate comfortable profit margins.[17]

Moreover, just before the trends in hospital care turned downward in the early 1980s, the for-profit chains took several steps in the direction of becoming fully integrated health delivery companies offering the entire range of health care services (sometimes in partnership with other organizations). The new ventures ranged from selling health insurance to operating health maintenance organizations (HMOs) and preferred-provider organizations (PPOs) and providing nursing home and home care.

Moreover, the for-profit chains did not remain passive once hospital use decreased and the reimbursement policies worsened. Their first move was to reassess the deployment of their assets, with the aim of reducing the size of facilities or withdrawing completely from activities in which the profit outlook had become unfavorable and redirecting their resources to areas where market opportunities appeared more promising.

The for-profit chains encountered greater difficulties than they had anticipated in the effort to transform themselves into integrated health service providers. Among some of the more egregious miscalculations were the marketing of health insurance, which turned out to be a more complex and costly undertaking than they had allowed for, and establishing walk-in clinics, which brought them into competition with local practitioners who often responded by not admitting patients to their hospitals. In most communities, the chains were a long way from having in place the range of facilities required to justify their claims to be fully integrated providers. Entrance into the HMO market also proved more complicated than they had expected, and it was unclear whether and to what extent expanded enrollment in HMOs would effectively increase (or perhaps decrease) the flow of patients into their hospitals. Finally, they seriously misjudged the time, financial resources, and managerial talent required to put together an integrated company.

The situation of the for-profit chains was threatened further as several of the larger health insurance companies moved into their competitive domain by also establishing and expanding HMOs. Although it is now uncertain whether any of these insurance company-sponsored HMOs will turn out to be long-term financial successes, the attempt of many underwriters to establish a major presence in this market has been another impediment to the hospital chains' pursuit of their strategies of integration. Their deep pockets notwithstanding, it now appears that several of the largest insurance companies are having second thoughts about remaining in the HMO market. Travelers and John Hancock, for instance, have indicated their plans to withdraw, and others are likely to follow.

Recent changes in the for-profit sector include, among other developments, the growing number of entrepreneurial efforts by small and medium-sized investors involved in the acquisition of hospitals, HMOs, imaging centers, clinics, and other facilities. Many of these investors are businessmen, whereas others are physicians; in some cases, businessmen and physicians organize joint ventures to which they contribute capital and professional leadership, respectively. Other new departures are cooperative arrangements by nonprofit institutions with for-profit chains; these range all the way from the University of Southern California's contract with National Medical Enterprises to erect a hospital on its campus to community hospitals that have joined with for-profit home care agencies to provide services for their discharged patients.

Urologists, neurologists, radiologists, and other specialists have established joint professional corporations which facilitate the purchase of expensive diagnostic and therapeutic equipment, often with multimillion dollar price tags, for use on a shared basis. Arnold Relman was an early critic of such entrepreneurial activities on the ground that they confront physicians with conflicts of interest in devising treatment plans for their patients.[18]

A reassessment of the for-profit hospital chains indicates that there is little basis for believing that their share of the total health care market will grow. Rather, the odds are that it will decline. Hospital Corporation of America (HCA) recently sold off more than half of its hospitals, containing about 40 percent of its total beds, to its former managers under a complex employee stock option plan that required large bank loans and ongoing financial support from HCA. The other large for-profit chains have also been pursuing aggressive scaling down and consolidation of strategies.

The for-profit sector does, however, face new opportunities when it comes to the inevitable expansion of nursing homes and other businesses related to the support and care of the increasing numbers of elderly persons, particularly those over 75 years of age. The Health Care Financing Administration (HCFA) projects that private funds for nursing home care will more than double between 1987 and 1995, from $21.8 billion to $47.1 billion.[19]

The more important finding implicit in these forecasts are the narrow margins for any meaningful tilting of the total health care system toward the for-profit sector. Of the $999.1 billion of total health expenditures projected for 1995, $423.5 billion is allocated to outlays by federal, state, and local governments. Of the remaining $575.6 billion of nongovernmental outlays, the hospital component is estimated to be $187.3 billion. It is unlikely that the for-profit chains will considerably increase their proportion of hospital revenue from their 1987 base; a share of 15 percent of hospital expenditures in 1995 for the for-profits would be liberal and would come to about $28 billion. If three-quarters of all private funds for nursing homes were allocated to the for-profit sector, that would add another $35 billion, making a total of $63 billion for institutional care in the for-profit sector. The long-established fields in which for-profit companies have dominated—drugs, eyeglasses and appliances, and program administration—contribute another $105 billion. Combining this sum with the $63 billion for institutional care and the $6 billion allocated to "other personal health care" brings the grand total of the for-profits to $174 billion.[20]

Data on expenditures for 1986 indicate a total for the for-profit sector—including drugs, medical equipment, hospital and nursing home care, program administration, and miscellaneous—of $101 billion, or 22 percent of the $458 billion.[21] The projected expenditures of $175 billion for the for-profit sector in 1995, out of nearly $1 trillion total, suggests that the share of the for-profit sector share is likely to decline.

The strongest of the for-profit chains continue to possess considerable financial strength, experienced managerial personnel, and entrepreneurial know-how that enable them to move quickly from unattractive situations into more promising markets. But it is difficult to see new opportunities within the health care arena that could assure them another decade of rapid growth and high profits. If their success is to continue, they will have to move beyond health care to a new sector of the economy.

This reassessment underscores the fact that the American people never came close to giving up their voluntary community hospitals and private medical practitioners for an investor-dominated, professional management structure whose goal has been the maximization of profit. Such a transformation would have required much more than short-term illusions on Wall Street and a pro-competition ideology run amok.

· 3 ·

American Medicine: The Power Shift

Americans try to foresee the future without taking the time or trouble to recall the past. But unless the past is placed in perspective, it is difficult to discover the shape and direction the future may take. Today the members of the medical profession and its leaders are disturbed about what the recent trends may portend for their work, their income, the well-being of their patients, and the structure of American medicine to come.

The reasons for the physicians' growing concern about the future will become clearer after I assess three distinct epochs of American medicine in this country: the era of physician domination, from the Flexner report in 1910 to the passage of Medicare in 1965; the era of the power shift, from 1966 to the end of 1984; and the problematic period that lies ahead when the medical profession will have one last opportunity to reassert its rights and exercise its responsibilities in helping to restructure American medicine.

The Era of Physician Domination

The Flexner report gave the American medical establishment an opportunity to control medical education and the supply of physicians. Soon afterward the American College of Surgeons moved aggressively to promulgate standards for the quality of hospital care, and the American Medical Association (AMA) devoted its efforts to the conditions of professional practice. The public agreed to this broad delegation of power to the medical profession on the assumption that in looking after its own interests the profession would improve the level of medical care.

In 1929, at the end of the prosperous 1920s, medicine accounted for a relatively small sector of the nation's economy: $3.5 billion of expenditures or about 3.5 percent of the gross national product. The large middle class was able to pay for its medical care while philanthropy and state governments, with major assistance from the donated services of the medical profession, were able to provide some medical care for the poor, especially those who lived in large cities. Although American medicine, particularly surgery, had made significant advances in the years following the Flexner report, its therapeutic armamentarium was still relatively limited in 1929.

At that time the profession of medicine, about which Lewis Thomas has written so perceptively, offered most practitioners a life of hard work and modest economic returns. The typical physician earned about two-and-a-half times the wages of a skilled worker. The public held most physicians in high esteem and was not envious or resentful of their earning power. In the depressed 1930s, the economic status of most physicians deteriorated along with the standard of living of almost all Americans. Young physicians often had to find interim employment as postal employees or taxi drivers and some borrowed the office of an established colleague during the evening hours in the hope of building a practice.

World War II was a watershed. Medicine made great strides with the advent of penicillin, advances in anesthesiology and surgery, and the broadening of medical education and consequent specialization. Fifteen million young Americans in the Armed Services and their dependents received excellent medical care. The Army lost only 6 percent of the battle casualties still alive when medical aid reached them. Quality medical care created, as the economists say, "a taste for medical care," which could be indulged after the war because of the increase in real income, the growth of hospital insurance, and the willingness of government to assist in the building of new hospitals (embodied in the Hill-Burton Act of 1946).

The medical establishment came out of World War II in a strong position. President Harry Truman twice submitted to Congress a proposal for National Health Insurance, an action that President Roosevelt had avoided when his administration drafted the Social Security legislation in 1935. But Truman's proposal faced strong opposition from the AMA and its powerful allies, particularly the leadership of the private sector. Although an increasing number of medical educators, politicians, and spokesmen for the public came out in favor of federal support for medical schools, the AMA was able to prevent federal legislation during the 1950s. Acute observers of the Washington scene believed that in matters that directly concerned them, the Catholic Church and the AMA were the two most successful lobbying organizations.

In the early 1960s, the AMA entered the fight over Medicare and it pulled out all the stops. It won some preliminary battles but lost the war. But it rallied from defeat and was able to force President Johnson to assure the medical profession that the Medicare regulations would not interfere with the established freedom of the physician-patient relationship. Neither signatory to this treaty understood that the new legislation would set the stage for a long-term acceleration of health care costs. And it was the response to these skyrocketing costs that came to play the dominant role in shifting the power center of American medicine away from physicians.

The Power Shift

Ten principal centers of power influence the structure of health care delivery. First is the *federal government.* In the year before Medicare's enactment in 1965, the total expenditure of the federal government for health care was approximately $5 billion, spent primarily to provide services to the Armed Forces and the Veterans Administration and to support biomedical research mainly through the National Institutes of Health. Health expenditures accounted for 1.8 percent of the federal budget. In 1984 total federal outlays for health exceeded $100-billion and accounted for over 11.5 percent of total federal outlays. Health expenditures have been rising more rapidly than any other item in the federal budget, not excepting defense. Small wonder that the administration and Congress are increasingly concerned with ways of constraining the rate of increase in health care expenditures, primarily for Medicare, which is by far the largest component of total federal outlays for health.

The next power center is the *government of the states*. States also have steeply rising health care costs. In the pre-Medicaid era they spent relatively modest sums for the care of the chronically ill, mostly mental patients, and for acute care for the poor. But for a decade before the passage of Medicaid, the states had begun to rely on new drugs to reduce the number of mental patients requiring in-patient care. Their responsibilities for tuberculosis patients had shrunk a decade earlier, in the 1950s.

In the mid-1980s the states were sharing with the federal government the costs of care for 22 million persons entitled to Medicaid at a cost to the states of $15-billion annually. In many states outlays for Medicaid represented the fastest growing item in their budgets. The *New York Times* reported that the states had resorted to 800 measures to slow Medicaid costs, including such draconian approaches as requiring physicians to request in advance permission to hospitalize a patient, setting stringent limits on the number of days of hospital care for which they would reimburse, freezing physician fees for 1985, and requiring families to contribute to nursing home care for their indigent relatives.

The third party that is reacting with vigor is the *business community*, particularly under the leadership of the recently formed business coalitions, which now number more than 200. Although large and small businesses have been long-term allies of organized medicine because of a shared belief that it was in their interests to keep government, particularly the federal government, out of health care, a major change has recently occurred. Business has become deeply concerned about the recent steep increases in its expenditures for health insurance for its employees, which in total amount is close to $100-billion annually.

For a long time, employers had responded positively to their workers' requests for broader and better insurance coverage, but in recent years they have recognized that health care costs are increasing at a rate considerably above inflation and they have had to seek ways to moderate their contributions. One employer survey indicated that about half of a representative group of middle-sized and large companies had altered their insurance plans between 1983 and 1985. Some shifted a part of their costs to their employees by introducing higher deductibles and copayments; others introduced measures aimed at controlling hospital utilization, such as claim reviews or requiring a second opinion prior to elective surgery.

The most dramatic instance of business concern has been the proposal of large employers in Arizona for a constitutional amendment aimed at placing the health care sector under a public-utility system of control. Since Arizona was the longtime holdout among the states with respect to joining Medicaid, this proposal is striking. Clearly, when ideology and profits conflict, American business is opting for new, even draconian, measures to slow health-related outlays.

The fourth power center is the *hospital system*. Until hospitals became big business—that is, until after the passage of Medicare and Medicaid—most of them were controlled by a volunteer board of directors who took their cues from the senior physicians on their staffs. As the inflow and outflow of dollars increased inordinately, hospital administrators dedicated to the growth of their institutions became a new center of influence, since the philanthropic contributions of their boards to help cover operating losses were no longer required. Government and insurance companies were providing more than 90 percent of the cash flow.

A few years ago there was a contretemps among the American Hospital Association (AHA), the AMA, and the two American Colleges (Physicians and Surgeons), about new policies by the Joint Commission on Accreditation of Hospitals (JCAH) governing appointment of nonphysicians to the hospital staff. Against the strenuous opposition of the two colleges, especially the American College of Surgeons, the JCAH decided that given the threat of antitrust action, it was better to revise the rules to facilitate the appointment of nonphysicians to hospital staffs.

Tension between the former close allies, physicians and hospitals, has also increased in other arenas. Many hospitals have been moving aggressively to vertical integration, that is, to delivering full services, including primary care, home care, and nursing home care. In the process they have started to compete with their own staffs and with other physicians. In turn, many physicians have begun to remove valuable diagnostic and therapeutic services out of the hospital to their offices or to other ambulatory-care settings that they control, thereby depriving hospitals of valuable sources of revenue. The acute care hospital, under increasing pressure in an environment of excess beds and reimbursement controls, no longer sees the physician as a reliable ally. And physicians in turn are looking askance at the marketing strategies of their hospitals.

A fifth new center of power is made up of the *insurance companies* that write group and individual health policies. In the past they primarily collected premiums and made payments to providers, with little authority or responsibility for determining either the fees of physicians or the efficiency and effectiveness with which hospitals used their resources. Recently, however, employers and governments that funnel funds through insurance companies have been pressing them to assume larger roles as monitors and controllers, namely, to pay out money only after they have ascertained that the expenditures are reasonable and that the providers acted prudently. No longer are insurance companies merely designers of new or modified plans, premium collectors, and bill payers.

A sixth center of influence resides in the *legal system* as it addresses the concept of acceptable quality care. In the search for culprits for accelerating costs, many physicians have identified lawyers as key factors because of the important role that they play in malpractice litigation. Contingency fee arrangements have unquestionably contributed to more and more litigation with a sharp upward drift in jury verdicts. The steeply rising costs of malpractice insurance have contributed to the cost acceleration; "defensive medicine" as a response to malpractice claims has added 10 to 15 percent to the nation's health bill.

It is questionable to single out lawyers as the major culprits. By action and inaction, physicians injure patients and occasionally cost them their lives. In our tradition, such patients or their heirs are entitled to seek judicial redress. In the post-Flexner era, American society turned over responsibility for setting standards of patient care to the medical profession, but despite its major accomplishments it was not able to establish and maintain tight controls. The AMA has indicated that as many as 10 percent of the medical professionals have disabilities (alcohol, drugs, mental instability) that interfere with the use of their skills. In a conference sponsored by the Council of Medical Specialty Societies (September 1984), William Curran of the Harvard Law School advised his audience that "physicians need to get back into the business of setting standards of care." The growth of malpractice suits reflects the extent to which physicians have increasingly lost control to lawyers and juries.

A seventh new power center is represented by *organized consumer groups*, among the most powerful of which is the American Association of Retired Persons (AARP) with a dues-paying membership of tens of millions. Many pages of the Association's magazine *Modern Maturity* are devoted to indictments of modern medicine, particularly the unconscionable rise in health care costs for the elderly. The AARP recommended that its members elicit opinions about health care from candidates for political office before casting their vote. Members were also urged to press Congress to pass legislation in favor of "assignment," which means that physicians treating Medicare beneficiaries must accept the federal government's payment as final.

Another new power center is the result of the rapid growth of *for-profit medical and hospital organizations,* including such big hospital chains as the Hospital Corporation of America, Humana, and American Medical International. In the mid-1980s these for-profit organizations accounted for about 10 percent of all inpatient acute care and were making significant inroads into the provision of ambulatory care, home care, and nursing home care. Although I do not anticipate that these and other for-profit providers such as Cigna and Prudential will ever dominate the health care market, given the strong tradition of nonprofit hospitals and the determination of many physicians to avoid employee status, for-profit enterprises represent a new and potent force in the shaping and reshaping of American medicine.

John Lister's article[1] about the growth of for-profit medicine in Great Britain is important in this context, especially in pointing out the insistence of the British medical leadership that physicians avoid conflicts between their professional responsibility to their patients and their economic self-interest. This is an issue that Relman has raised on occasion and that needs reemphasis.

Still another power center can be identified as the "Guadalajara syndrome." The large numbers of U.S. citizens who are studying medicine abroad, in Mexico, the Caribbean, the Philippines, and Europe, have every intention of returning to this country for their clerkships and residency training with the aim of entering the mainstream of American medicine. Many decisions that should be made about enrollments in U.S. medical schools and specialty training will be affected by the strong pressures exerted on behalf of this sizable pool of off-shore students. There is little point for Congress and state legislatures to cut back on undergraduate and graduate medical education without antecedent or concomitant action aimed at reducing and eliminating the inflow of physicians trained abroad.

The tenth shift in power is occurring in *the national political arena.* The Senate debated for only forty minutes before it enacted legislation authorizing diagnosis-related groups (DRGs— prospective payments to hospitals by diagnosis). The AMA was alone in its opposition, except for support from the AFL-CIO. All the other constituencies favored the new approach. Small wonder that a leading member of the Senate later remarked that he no longer found it necessary to heed the wishes of the AMA.

The shift in power in American medicine can be encapsulated as follows: the medical profession can no longer count on its erstwhile allies—hospitals, business, insurance companies—to keep the government at arm's length in making decisions that affect health care. All of these power constituencies, and several others including organized consumer groups, are determined to slow the advance in health care costs. Physicians are no longer the sole arbiters.

Future Control

It would be a misreading of the foregoing, however, to conclude that the medical establishment, which has suffered a serious erosion of its power, has limited say in decisions regarding health care. Far from it. Survey results attest to the fact that the American public continues to hold their personal physicians in high esteem, far above the respect they have for most leaders, governmental and corporate. Of course the public wants health care costs to be controlled. But it has not chosen, surely not at this point, to take the future control of health care away from the medical profession and to entrust it to businessmen, bureaucrats, economists, and planners.

The question about what happens next is moot. If the medical profession can reach a consensus and if its leadership can agree about a broad front of critical issues, it can regain much of its earlier power and influence, which it needs to shape the future of the system.

But it can recapture the ground it has lost only if it can formulate sensible and sound policy recommendations on a large number of contentious issues, most of which lie beyond the ken of the lay community. For example, the leadership must talk to the issue of the future supply of physicians. As the *Wall Street Journal* reported, most of the European members of the Organization for Economic Cooperation and Development have a physician glut that is having an adverse effect on the quality of medical care. Underemployed and unemployed physicians are a menace to the public's health as well as to its pocketbooks. Many explanations for silence on this critical issue, including fear of antitrust prosecution, are offered by medical leaders. But it is ludicrous that the public has received little guidance from the profession to date on this critical issue.

Similarly, Congress is edging up to enacting major changes in the financing of graduate medical education. It is highly unlikely that Congress will continue the liberal pass-through to teaching hospitals. But Congress needs the best advice it can get from the medical leadership about the number and types of residency places that should be provided and preferred methods for financing them. For years, informed observers have believed that the costs of graduate medical education should not be paid for by hospitalized patients.

Another critical area in which the public needs advice and guidance from the medical profession is new technology, the conditions under which it should be introduced, and whether or not it should be routinely reimbursable by third-party payers. Several years ago much excitement was generated by computerized axial tomography machines, or CAT scanners, and the conditions under which hospitals should be allowed to purchase them. It seemed to me at the time, and even more so in retrospect, that the medical leadership failed to say with one loud voice that the CAT scan represented the most important advance in noninvasive imaging in the history of diagnostic medicine and that the capital and operating costs were well within the capacity of the nation to underwrite. But this is not a blanket endorsement of all new technology nor of third-party reimbursement for it. We need demonstrations and assessments before expensive new technology is incorporated into prevailing patterns of practice. And the public looks to the medical profession to lead such assessments.

American medicine is reaching a major turning point in its evolution. The passage of Medicare and the consequent cost inflation that is still largely uncontrolled has led to the emergence of new and powerful groups that insist on having their say about the restructuring of the health care system—government, business, insurance companies, and organized consumer groups, to mention only the more important. The question is whether the medical profession, whose leaders have been muted in recent years, will reassert itself and talk loudly and clearly about issues of major concern to itself, the American people, and the future of American medicine.

But if its counsel is to carry weight, the medical leadership must not be overly concerned about maintaining the above-average incomes of physicians, which increased in the post-World War II period from two-and-a-half to five-and-a-half times the earnings of a skilled worker. Rather, it should proffer advice directed toward assuring that American medicine will remain in the forefront of the developed world; that appropriate steps be taken to assure strong research and development activities; that the health care system be accessible to all, rich and poor alike; and that it can operate in an efficient and effective manner with due respect for the general welfare. If, and only if, the medical leadership responds in this wise will it be able to retain and enhance the esteem in which the public still holds the profession, and only then will its voice be accorded the respect it requires to lead in the restructuring of our health care system.

Privatization of Health Care

The term *privatization*, while not commonly used in discussions of policy issues, is generally equated with activities that are carried out in the private sector. This is a simple, but not necessarily clarifying definition. It gives rise to the following questions. Can the U.S. economy be divided into two sectors, private and public? This is questionable, given the size and importance of the nonprofit sector,[1] which accounts for not less than 8 percent of employment and gross national product (GNP).[2] What is included in the concept of "activities carried out" in a specific sector? Does it relate to management, financing, sales, or to the totality of these functions? How does one distinguish between private and nonprivate or preferably, between for-profit and not-for-profit (government and nonprofit), in the case of health care in the United States? Government (all levels—federal, state, and local) is responsible for financing 42 percent[3] of the half a trillion dollar system (1987 estimate)[4] but it produces and delivers a far smaller proportion of the total output. Conversely, how should one categorize the hospital sector with annual expenditures of over $200 billion for care that is performed predominantly by nonprofit institutions[5] whose primary sources of payment are government and the private for-profit sector (corporate insurance)?

To all these considerations we should add the more subtle but nevertheless critically important public-private intermingling that is found in the several phases of biotechnology—from initial laboratory research, through development and production, to ultimate utilization or application in the provision of medical care. Some 85 percent of all funding for basic biomedical research is provided by the federal government, primarily through the National Institutes of Health (NIH); almost all of the development and manufacturing of the technological armamentarium of modern medicine is performed under the aegis of the private (for-profit) sector; and most of the major advances in technology are actually used in hospitals that are predominantly nonprofit institutions.

The Pre-World War II Health Care Enterprise

The relevance of this lengthy excursus on the place of the health care sector in the U.S. economy is a consequence of the ideological orientation of the Reagan administration, with its professed admiration for private enterprise and its antagonism toward the role of government in virtually all of its civilian functions. One of its early spokesmen, David Stockman, the former director of the Office of Management and Budget, stated that medical care in the United States had historically been characterized by competitive markets.[6] This amounted to historical revisionism. In point of fact, all through this century and, in the case of major urban centers, the preceding century as well, the predominant institution in the U.S. health care sector has been the community hospital, heavily financed by philanthropic contributions and governed by a voluntary board of trustees chosen from among the leaders of the community.

Although U.S. physicians have been strongly wedded to the fee-for-service mode of practice, it would be a serious mistake to overlook—certainly for the period prior to World War II—the extent to which they had a foot in the nonprofit sector as well. Private practitioners treated many patients for less than the customary fee or for no fee and devoted significant blocks of time to unpaid, voluntary service in clinics and on the wards of hospitals.

At the outbreak of World War II, medicine was a relatively minor segment of the U.S. economy. The affluence of the American medical profession dates only from the 1950s.[7] Earlier, most physicians had modest earnings, in the $5,000 range, and philanthropic funds played a critical role in providing the capital and covering the deficits of community hospitals.[8] To be sure, a considerable governmental plant provided acute care, mostly for the poor, and chronic care for TB and psychiatric patients. Withal, many of the rural poor, and particularly the blacks, had little or no access to the system. A minority of the nation's hospitals were proprietary institutions, most of them owned and operated by physicians. Most medical schools were constituent bodies of public or private (nonprofit) universities; in addition, there was a residual number of nonprofit, independent medical colleges. Finally, foundations were important funders of medical research.

By no stretch of the imagination nor even of ideology could the U.S. health care system at the outset of World War II be said to have been a predominantly—and surely not exclusively— private, for-profit enterprise.

The Post-World War II Transformation

The surest way to delineate the magnitude of the transformation of the U.S. health care system since World War II is to note that in 1950 total expenditures came to approximately $13.5 billion or 4.7 percent of GNP.[9] The comparable figures for 1987 are $500 billion or 11.2 percent of a much larger GNP. Since our focus is on privatization, we will call attention to several critical policy decisions that served to move the system in the direction of privatization or away from it.

More by accident than intent, health care insurance as an employee benefit was vastly expanded during World War II, following a ruling by the War Labor Board that such benefits were not in violation of the wartime wage freeze. Some years after the war, the Bureau of Internal Revenue ruled that employer contributions for health insurance were a legitimate business expense and thus not subject to tax; the value of the benefit to the employee was similarly tax exempt. Alain Enthoven has estimated that in 1986 the total value of these tax expenditures approximated $49 billion.[10] Over the years, Blue Cross-Blue Shield (a nonprofit organization until the tax reform legislation of 1986) and commercial carriers have divided the health insurance market which currently yields almost $140 billion in annual premiums.[11] The business remained in private hands; the

Congress twice rejected the recommendation of President Harry Truman to pass a national health insurance bill.

Despite sizable expansions of the Veterans Administration and the Armed Services health care systems, the role of government as a deliverer of care has declined as a consequence of the closure of TB hospitals, the marked reduction (over 75 percent) in the census of state mental hospitals, and most recently, the closure or sale of a considerable number of local, county, and state acute care hospitals. The enactment of Medicare and Medicaid in 1965, however, substantially increased (by about one third) government's share of the total health bill; this is exclusive of its tax expenditure contribution.

The regulatory role of government has increased substantially over the last third of a century, a function that has persisted despite the distaste of the Reagan administration for regulation and bureaucratic oversight.[12] The introduction in 1983 of prospective, per case reimbursement to hospitals by Medicare inevitably involved the federal government in yearly rate-setting negotiations with the hospital industry; since then Congress has established a commission to consider changes in the payment system for physicians who treat Medicare beneficiaries. In addition, the PROs have the task of assessing the quality of care that providers offer Medicare patients. While some states have eliminated their certificate of need requirements, others have not. And an increasing number of states are testing different mechanisms for providing coverage for the large number of uninsured persons. While the introduction of the prospective payment system was aimed at broadening the scope of the market in setting hospital rates, there is no evidence that the total weight of government regulation has declined.

The postwar years witnessed an almost hundredfold increase in total funding for biomedical research, from $161 million in 1950 to over $14 billion in 1986, with government, principally the federal government, accounting for more than half; the corporate sector is the other major funder.[13] States and the federal government were the principal sectors responsible for the large-scale expansion of medical schools, which doubled the nation's output of physicians between 1965 and 1980.[14] Through the passage of the Hill-Burton Act in 1946, the federal government made available substantial funds for the construction of hospitals (and later other types of health care facilities) in underbuilt and underserved areas of the country. The federal government and the states also made it easier and cheaper for nonprofit hospitals to borrow money for building, expansion and renovation.

One can summarize the foregoing disparate trends in the four decades after World War II as follows:

(1) The United States unequivocally rejected a comprehensive system of national health insurance. It was willing, however, to go part of the way to insure health care for the elderly and provide federal-state support for the categorically poor (welfare recipients) and others whose incomes were close to the poverty line.

(2) The United States relied on the private sector (employers) to provide insurance benefits for workers and usually for their dependents as well. The federal government assisted by granting tax exemption for such insurance contributions.

(3) Both the federal government and the private sector vastly increased their funding for biomedical research and development. Most of the federal dollars, however, were awarded to members of academic institutions on the basis of a competitive peer review system.

(4) Ever since the early 1970s there has been growing restiveness on the part of the federal government and state governments, and more recently the corporate sector as well, with the relentlessly rising trends in health care costs. In the face of a public that favors greater, not smaller, expenditure for health care, however, the dominant payers (government and industry, which together cover about 70 percent of the total bill) have had little success in their multiple efforts at cost containment.[15]

A Closer Look at Privatization

There is little in the foregoing review of post-World War II developments to support the contention that the U.S. health care system is far advanced on the road to privatization. The clearest evidence to the contrary is the fact that government accounts for around 42 percent of total expenditures; the remaining 58 percent is provided by consumers and employers in roughly equal proportions. But if one factors in government's contribution in the form of tax expenditures, its share approximates half of all outlays.

There are other reasons for caution not to exaggerate the extent to which private sector forces dominate the U.S. health care system. In effect, consumers pay less than 30 percent of health care costs out of pocket; the remaining 30 percent of nongovernmental expenditure represents payments made by insurance. No one would contend that an individual who is covered by insurance makes his expenditure decisions just as he would if the funds were coming from his own pocket. In this connection, we have noted that the proportion of public dollars has been increasing, not declining. In short, while the U.S. health care system has been "monetarized," it has not been privatized, surely not as of the present.[16]

Is Privatization the Wave of the Future?

The growing currency of the concept of the privatization of the U.S. health care system is not simply the creation of Reagan ideology and the imposition of a per case, prospective payment system of Medicare reimbursement that provides greater scope for price competition among deliverers of care. Other signs also suggest that the health care market may be moving in the direction of privatization. We will consider the most conspicuous of these developments.

The surge of the for-profit hospital chains in the 1970s and early 1980s had to attract attention not only among speculators and investors on Wall Street who were willing to fuel this growth, but also among the public at large. The dramatic expansion of the major chains appeared to present a major challenge to the U.S. hospital structure, which had long been dominated by the nonprofit community hospital. This initial success led some analysts, notably Paul Ellwood, to forecast that the entire system would soon be preempted by ten to twenty Super-Meds. Yet, in the short span of three years—1984–1987—the prospects of the chains have plummeted. Rather than continue to acquire hospitals, they are seeking to dispose of many that they now possess. Their profits have suffered steep declines. Investors have turned cautious. Not even their managements still believe that the future will be theirs.[17]

The last two decades have seen one of the bastions of American capitalism—the insurance industry—extend its sphere of activities from health care underwriting to service delivery, primarily through the establishment of for-profit HMOs. Such movement surely points to the expansion of private sector activities. Nevertheless, one must not exaggerate the extent of their involvement. It is unlikely that the HMOs operated by the major insurance companies have enrolled more than 15 percent of the total national HMO membership of 21 million. The latter figure approximates 10 percent of the U.S. population. Some analysts believe that the recent steep gains in HMO enrollments will continue until they encompass 50 percent or more of the population. My guess is that they will have a hard time reaching the 25 percent mark, competing as they do with many alternative systems of managed care that allow patients greater choice of physicians.

A considerable number of physician-entrepreneurs have joined with other physicians, with the hospitals at which they work or others, or with medical supply companies (often involving leasing arrangements) to establish an ambulatory clinic, an imaging center, a rehabilitation or wellness institute or some other types of specialized treatment centers. These developments indicate advancing privatization; nevertheless, at this point in time, it is hard to anticipate that the totality of these entrepreneurial efforts by physicians will lead to more than a marginal shift in the extant structure.

More important by far than these physicians' organizations are the efforts of nonprofit hospitals to restructure themselves along lines that will enable them to engage in for-profit activities in the field of health care as well as in other fields. Worried about their long-run financial viability, they see advantages to expansion, diversification, joint ventures, and much more. Institutions with strong management and access to capital are likely to find one or more profitable niches. Many others, weaker in managerial or financial resources, are likely to discover that making money is not very easy, especially for the inexperienced. Several recent initiatives by for-profit organizations appeared to be part of rapidly advancing privatization. A few years ago the big for-profit chains seemed about to acquire a considerable number of academic health centers (AHCs). In point of fact, four AHCs were acquired by the chains. Since then there has been no further action on this front nor is there likely to be, given the more vulnerable balance sheets of the for-profit groups.

Humana, one of the most aggressive of the chains, stole the limelight several years ago when it recruited the renowned cardiac surgeon, William DeVries, from the University of Utah to head a newly established artificial heart implantation program at a Humana hospital in Louisville, Kentucky, its corporate headquarters. Humana then agreed to subsidize the costs for an initial group of patients who, DeVries believed, could profit from surgery. For months Humana, the staff, and the patients all but monopolized the media, but now this medical drama has faded from view. The public must have had some second thoughts about the quality of life of the patients who had undergone the implantation and about the value of the short incremental period of life they gained. How much Humana actually profited from this initiative, over and above the unmatched publicity, is uncertain. Inpatient operating data for its hospitals indicate declines in tandem with the rest of the proprietary hospital sector, and the company is in the process of disposing of its HMOs which had achieved an enrollment of 350,000.[18]

An even more unconventional departure has been the establishment in the state of Tennessee of a for-profit hospital that specializes in the treatment of cancer victims for whom it develops biological and chemical substances specific to each individual patient's pathology. The cost per patient is reputed to be around $35,000 for a course of treatment. Here is a situation combining applied research, development, and treatment all under a for-profit umbrella. There has been no report of the replication of this enterprising departure, which was of sufficient interest to the medical profession to be the subject of two articles in *The New England Journal of Medicine*.[19]

In sum, the foregoing examples—and they could easily be multiplied—point to the presence of forces at work indicative of the increasing privatization of the U.S. health care system. But individually and collectively they do not add up to a strong movement. Privatization does not appear to be the wave of the future.

A Concluding Note

A few economists, in particular Kenneth Arrow, Robert Evans, and I, are convinced that the paradigm of the competitive market cannot be applied to health care, surely not in an affluent economy in which insurance plays a major role.[20] Accordingly, I see no prospect for further large-scale privatization of the U.S. health care system beyond its current level—the 60, 50, or 30 percent mark depending on the criterion that is used: insurance plus consumer out-of-pocket payments, direct governmental outlays plus tax expenditures, or solely consumer out-of-pocket payments.

I see two alternative scenarios for the period up to the year 2000. If the U.S. (and world) economies do not suffer a serious recession, the odds are that the present ratios of private to public will continue to prevail. In the event that the U.S. economy falters, I believe that the increasingly fragile private insurance system will not survive the strain and that the country will move to some form of federal-state insurance system that will cover hospital and catastrophic care for all. In that event, we will be in retreat from the current level of privatization.

· 5 ·

High-Tech Medicine

Historical Perspective

When things go wrong with the functioning of a major societal system, as they did with the U.S. economy in the 1930s, the search is on for a culprit. At the time one group identified "technology" as responsible for the persistent double digit unemployment. The continuing rise of health expenditures as a percentage of GNP over the last two decades has led prominent politicians, academicians, and health care analysts not only to place the blame on high-tech but to insist that the nation will soon face the dilemma of rationing such care to the elderly or confronting the financial collapse of the health care system.

This chapter reviews the multitudinous forces that have brought high-tech to center stage in the U.S. health care system and explores whether the system is in danger of being bankrupted by technology's unremitting advances. The better we understand the process that has resulted in the dominant role of high-tech in contemporary medical care, the less likely we will be to misjudge its potency and exaggerate its potential to undermine the financing of our health care system. Health policy is sufficiently complex without the confusion that comes of chasing phantasmagoria.

When Abraham Flexner published his report on the restructuring of American medical education in 1910, the major countries of Western Europe were well on their way to broadening and deepening the scientific basis for medical diagnosis and therapy. Flexner was convinced that if the United States was not to fall behind in medical practice it had no option but to establish roots in the mainstream of scientific inquiry and benefit from the continuing advances in biology, chemistry, physiology, and the other core disciplines. Physicians, educated and trained in basic and applied science, would be better prepared to treat and cure their patients.

The rapid decline of proprietary medical schools and the absorption of most surviving medical schools within the university complex established the preconditions for science-based medicine. The full-time professors of medicine became the first exemplars of high-tech medicine. Their raison d'être was to push back the frontiers of knowledge and in the process strengthen the foundation for practice.

A second force that added momentum to this scientific-technological trend was the post-World War I elaboration of a strengthened pharmaceutical industry that invested increasing amounts of stockholders' money in developing new and improved drugs and related agents. In 1940, industry's annual investment in biomedical research and development (R&D) accounted for more than half of the national total of $45 million, a small part of which it made available to the medical schools for drug testing and related research.

World War II and its aftermath provided the breakthrough that catapulted high-tech medicine into a position of dominance. The revolution in antibiotics dates from the late 1930s, and the period of active hostilities during the war saw many advances in surgery, the uses of blood, psychiatry, rehabilitative medicine and others. The war's influence on public attitudes toward enlarged expenditures for health care was truly momentous. The passage of the Hill-Burton Act in 1946, for example, ensured that many rural and small communities would soon boast a local hospital, the emerging center of modern medical practice. And the Congress moved to underwrite biomedical research at ever larger amounts. In 1940 total federal expenditures for biomedical R&D amounted to $3 million, overwhelmingly for intramural programs. In 1965 federal outlays were slightly under $1.2 billion, a 400-fold increase. Most of the funding went to the nation's leading medical schools.

These large annual federal appropriations not only created a new cadre of well-funded research professors at the leading

AHCs, but also provided money for new research laboratories and equipment and underwrote the training of specialists and sub-specialists, some of whom joined the growing numbers of well-trained researchers.

The preexisting balance of power in the medical school was radically altered. The clinicians ceded their preeminence to the laboratory researchers who were able to attract large federal funds, expand their staffs, and concentrate their efforts on pushing back the biomedical frontiers. One byproduct of this realignment was the impetus it provided for accelerating the trend toward specialization. And the increased number and proportion of specialists and sub-specialists helped to assure the victory of high-tech medicine. Each specialty and sub-specialty recognized the value of developing unique diagnostic and therapeutic procedures—keys to greater prestige and income. The new federal largesse for biomedical research accelerated the rate of expansion. If the medical schools had had to depend on university budgets for expanding their research, their progress would have been much slower. Similarly, absent outside funding, the medical faculties would never have trained so many specialists and sub-specialists with their enthusiasm for technical advances and sophisticated interventions.

Why were politicans not only willing but eager to make ever larger appropriations for biomedical research? The answer is simple and straightforward. The public was pressing for cures, sooner rather than later, to the many dread diseases, in particular heart disease, cancer, and stroke, which together accounted for the majority of all deaths. Moreover, the substantial and sustained growth of the U.S. economy between 1945 and 1965 made it relatively easy for the Congress to find the additional money required to keep increasing the funding for research. In years of budgetary surpluses, there is nothing that politicians prefer more than appropriating additional money for good causes, such as biomedical research, which enjoy enthusiastic public support. Even in years of financial stringency, Congress has tended to appropriate more funds for biomedical research than presidents, Republican or Democratic, have requested.

The media have contributed and continue to contribute to the public's interest in and appreciation of high-tech medicine. Just recall the coverage that Humana received when it sought to prolong the lives of selected patients through the use of the artificial heart. In my judgment then, and even more so now, Humana's involvement with the broadcasting companies in reporting on the treatment of these patients was a questionable business tactic since the odds from the outset were for an unfavorable outcome. Some marketing experts believe, however, that additional brand recognition is good, no matter how achieved. The enlarged space that the daily newspapers have been directing to health affairs, including items on esoteric research projects, also speaks to the heightened interest of the public.

Important as the leadership of the medical profession, politicians, the public, and the press have been in advancing the role of high-tech medicine, note must also be taken of the influence of private sector enterprises, primarily pharmaceutical and medical equipment companies, whose principal and often sole market are hospitals, physicians, and patients. Although our domestic pharmaceutical industry expanded after World War I, its period of explosive growth came in the aftermath of the second World War, fueled by the accelerated national expenditures for health care and biomedical research. With over 1,000 companies engaged in the manufacture of drugs, having an annual shipment value in the $40 billion range, U.S.-based pharmaceutical companies are clearly important players in the health care arena. When one notes that in 1987 the pharmaceutical and related industries spent almost $6.5 billion on R&D (mostly D) to bring new products and services to the market, it is obvious what significant players they have become: their total annual spending for R&D approximates the outlays of the federal government.

But there is more to private sector initiatives. One must also take into account the almost 3,000 medical instrument and supply companies with a total shipment value about half the pharmaceutical output, circa $20 billion. In these two major industry sectors powerful forces operate to advance high-tech. Just consider the large number of detail men who are out on the road calling on physicians with samples of their old and particularly their new products, and the special sales forces that are employed to interest hospitals and other health institutions in purchasing equipment that, in the case of magnetic resonance imaging (MRI) or positron emission tomography (PET) can entail initial outlays of $2 to $4 million a unit. Not to be overlooked in this connection is the strength of the producing companies which include some of the world's largest and most powerful multinationals, such as General Electric and Siemens.

The pursuit of profits by strong private sector companies is a generic phenomenon, not distinctive or unique to the health care sector. What is different, however, are the forces that play on the prospective purchaser. Up to World War II, and to a lesser degree up to the passage of Medicare and Medicaid, the amount of new equipment that hospitals could acquire was limited by the amount of philanthropic capital that they were able to raise. This was a powerful restraining factor.

All this changed: hospitals succeeded in obtaining reimbursement for depreciation; third party payers, after 1965, covered over 90 percent of their total expenditures; nonprofit hospitals gained access to the private bond market, and the for-profits were able to tap the equity markets. The post-1965 era witnessed the explosive growth of high-tech. Potential customers were no longer strapped for money, and producers were able to offer them an array of new and improved technologies of which the revolution in imaging was only the most dramatic.

Hospitals have always competed with each other, not so much on price as on their ability to attract and retain the more prominent physicians in their community. In turn, physicians have been attracted to the staffs of institutions that are in the best position to provide them access to cutting-edge technology and strong support services.

Several additional forces contributed to the sweeping victory of high-tech medicine. Third party payers—commercial insurance, the Blues, and government—with minor exceptions have recognized as eligible for reimbursement any new procedure or service that gains the approval of the medical profession. By way of exercising restraint, the most that the third party payers were inclined to do was to delay, usually for only a short period of time, a new treatment modality requiring expensive new technology. Certificate of need legislation by the federal government and selected states did relatively little to slow the advance of new technology. True, hospitals faced additional barriers in making large capital investments, but in many instances clinics and physician groups were able to circumvent these barriers. Once the evidence began to accumulate that the new technology could contribute to the quality of care, its diffusion was well nigh assured.

In response to the multiple breakthroughs in molecular biology and biotechnology, venture capitalists have become increasingly interested in health care, not least because of the present and potential scale of the market. Hospitals currently spend about $200 billion annually and the forecasts by HCFA are for very rapid increases by 1995, continuing to 2000.

Closely related but still distinguishable from the role that venture capitalists in the United States are playing to narrow the time between discoveries in the laboratory and the marketing of new products and services is the increasing globalization of companies engaged in medical product innovation. The Swiss have long had a strong presence in the American pharmaceutical market and one can point to strong niche positions by companies based in the United Kingdom, Sweden, Germany, Israel, and others.

The above identification of the principal forces propelling high-tech medicine must be supplemented by reference to the human resources factor. The leading research-oriented ACHs have set the pace for U.S. medicine. The specialist societies have become the center of primary interest to most practicing physicians. And able young people contemplating medical research as a career have been strongly influenced by the large number of American Nobel Laureates in medicine and physiology.

Is High-Tech a Threat?

The conventional wisdom about high-tech medicine is full of ambiguities and confusions. For example, we were warned years ago by Lewis Thomas that most of what we call high-tech is really "half-way" technology that does not provide definitive understanding of the causes of our most destructive diseases and the reasons for our less than constructive interventions. Although Thomas emphasizes that we expect too much from contemporary medicine, that we devote too many resources to it, and that input/output ratios for many costly procedures are distressingly low and often negative, he sees no option for our society other than to continue down the road that we are on and look forward to the time when biological research will provide definitive answers to the problems that now confront us. Technology will, in his view, pay off but only in the indefinite future.

When the CAT scanner first appeared there was selected opposition to its broad diffusion on the ground that every patient who presented with a headache would be scanned and that the costs of the new equipment were beyond the capacity of the health care system to absorb. Both objections seemed to me to be wide of the mark. The fact that a new technology may be misused is a commonplace. And the costs of new technologies tend to fall once demand expands. The critical question that I put at the time to one of the nation's leading radiologists who had been brainwashed by his economist colleagues was whether the CAT scanner was a significant advance in imaging. He replied that it was the most important advance in imaging since the X-ray and that it was completely noninvasive. His assessment convinced me that discussions about cost would prove largely irrelevant and this in fact turned out to be the case.

Clearly, considerations of cost cannot be ignored when it comes to the purchase of CT, MRI, PET and still other esoteric imaging devices, but the point to be emphasized is the need for making room in a half-trillion-dollar health care system for new technology that promises significant gains in diagnosis and therapy. Other facets of the technology-cost relationship are frequently misperceived. The general view among economists is that technological improvements are the key to economic growth. New and improved methods of producing and distributing goods and services are the source of productivity gains. Many students of health affairs have been distressed, however, by the fact that technology in the health arena appears to be cost-enhancing, not cost-reducing. But that is an error in analysis, not an exception to the generalization. The error stems from the fact that the output measure has been incorrectly specified. It makes little sense to compare a Ford automobile of 1930 with the most recent vintage. How much more irrelevant is comparing the effectiveness of a day's hospitalization, or a specific procedure such as an appendectomy, then and now. In the mid-1920s the average length of stay for a routine appendectomy was of the order of two weeks, while today it is more like four days. Because of limited diagnostic capabilities many were operated on for appendicitis who today would be treated medically. Moreover, in the earlier day many who were operated on developed infections which resulted in extended hospitalization. And not a few failed to survive the operation. If the output is grossly undervalued, there is no way to judge the productivity of new technological inputs.

A related doctrine, popular among economists, was first formulated by William Baumol. Known as "the cost disease," it emphasizes the ineluctable increase in the costs of services relative to goods, as a consequence of the heavy dependence of services on human resource inputs while goods production can take advantage of cost reductions inherent in labor-saving technology. Once again, the generalization doesn't hold up: there have been very heavy capital investments in many service sectors and the labor component of total hospital expenditures has declined in the last two decades from about two-thirds to one-half.

However one evaluates the "cost disease" proposition, it is important to emphasize that technological advances in diagnosis and therapy often require the deployment of additional skilled personnel. Anyone who has been present at an open-heart procedure is struck by the large supporting staff, each of whom has a critical role in assuring a satisfactory outcome.

The critics of high-tech medicine come from diverse groups. Some are concerned that our society should not spend so much on improving health care, given the demands for other critical investments, from improved education to a more protected environment. Others believe that a shift from high-tech therapeutics to preventive services would be desirable. Still others, notably John Wennberg, Robert Brook, and William Knaus, while not opposed to high tech, believe that it is being overused and misused and that greater professional leadership and control could effect substantial dollar savings and gains in patient outcomes. In the face of so many different strictures about high-tech medicine, the clarification of public policy is at best a complex undertaking; at worst clarification may be long delayed.

Open Issues

There is a growing presumption among physicians, the public, and medical ethicists that the technological imperative has presented our contemporary health care system with one overriding challenge: the ability to prolong human life without providing a tolerable quality of life for the patient whose days or years have been extended. Legislators, courts, and the medical establishment have moved a considerable distance to broaden choices for patients or their surrogates to avoid such prolongation of life in the absence of any functionality, as in the case of persons in a permanent vegetating state. It may be some time before the United States follows the practice of The Netherlands and permits, under various safeguards, the use of euthanasia, but we are definitely on the way to setting bounds on the use of high-tech medicine for patients who cannot be restored to a minimum of human functioning.

The most contentious issue on the agenda of certain critics of high tech is the urgent need that our society faces to limit access to high-tech interventions for the elderly on the grounds that we cannot afford to provide to all who could benefit interventions that cost $150,000, such as a liver transplant and the requisite postoperative maintenance drugs. These analysts believe that the rationing of high-tech medicine is inevitable and the sooner we face the challenge the better.

Following this line President Nixon warned the nation in 1970, when health expenditures amounted to $75 billion and accounted for 7.5 percent of the GNP, that the United States was facing an economic crisis because of the acceleration in its health care costs. In 1987 the comparable figures were $498 billion and 11.2 percent of the GNP. Many economists are justifiably worried about the state of the U.S. economy because of the combined budget and balance of payments deficits, but surely not because of the high level of health care outlays. Indeed, the one major confrontation that the Congress faced involving a significant life-prolonging therapy, renal dialysis, led to legislation that made it broadly available to all.

The transplant issue has been contained to date by the relative paucity of available organs. In the event that organs become more readily available and particularly if artificial organs are perfected to a point where they prove to be good substitutes, then the high cost of transplantation may require the public to look anew at the question of rationing. But until the time when financial pressures force the issue, the American people are likely to insist that high tech be available to all.

The limited economic resources of the individual or the hospital where he or she is being treated have long resulted in *de facto* rationing. But that is inevitable in a society such as ours with a wide dispersion of family income and institutional capabilities. Despite such *de facto* rationing, the priority issue is whether our democratic society should move to a system of *de jure* rationing and whether age is the appropriate criterion.

Concluding Observations

The thrust of this analysis has been to underscore that high-tech medicine is the only game in town. Even its most severe critics go no further than to suggest modest modifications such as reducing our expectations for "half-way" technologies while pressing ahead with medical research, strengthening the existing methods and improving technological assessments to assure that costly new investments are justified, or restructuring the scope of high tech through rationing so as to keep the total health budget from escalating out of hand.

The two approaches aimed at controlling high-tech innovations, rationing aside, are directed first to putting in place a strong technological assessment mechanism aimed at weighing the potential gains of a new technology before its diffusion is approved. Congress walked up to this problem a few years ago and ultimately walked away from it by supporting the formation of a multi-interest review body under the aegis of the Institute of Medicine of the National Academy of Sciences. Such an effort is now under way, but with severely constricted funding it is far from clear that it has been or will be able to affect the rate of diffusion except at the margin.

The point is worth making, because it is so frequently overlooked, that new technology does not emerge in a single burst of creative innovation but rather follows a process in which the early models are highly imperfect and become refined and more effective over time as a result of the efforts of many different individuals and groups. Consideration of this fact together with the multi-year periods required to launch and carry through controlled clinical trials, often with ambiguous or at least not definitive results, reinforces the inherent limitations of a strong technological assessment mechanism. Pushed to the extreme one could argue that putting such a mechanism in place, if it were possible to do so (itself problematic), would be dysfunctional.

The second approach is geared to putting in place a review mechanism that would continuously evaluate the appropriateness of various diagnostic and therapeutic procedures from the vantage of an expanding knowledge base, both laboratory and clinical. The RAND Corporation has taken the lead in recent years to explore such an approach and preliminary review findings suggest that a number of procedures performed by physicians are questionable or counterindicated.

One can accept the reviewers' judgments about the sizable "overuse" of these selected procedures without agreeing with the recommendations of the RAND analysts that such procedures should be performed at only a limited number of sites (major teaching centers) subjected to continuous evaluation. Some of the unanswered questions about the proposed RAND solution aimed at improving patient outcomes and at the same time reducing total health care expenditures are as follows. To what extent can any evaluative procedure do more than differentiate the "erroneous" use of a procedure from the more usual category of "questionable judgment?" How many such evaluative studies, often requiring multi-year investigations, can the 20 to 40 major research-oriented AHCs undertake and carry through to a definitive conclusion? What sanctions can be exercised and by whom in the case of physicians who decide in their best judgment not to follow the guidelines that emerge from completed studies? And more to the point, what happens in the many months-to-years while the studies are under way? One can add to this list the issue of the additional costs of forcing many patients to travel to distant sites for possible treatment; the relevance of the findings in a highly dynamic therapeutic environment in which new approaches surpass old ones; and the possibility of easier, less expensive, and more effective mechanisms such as the refusal by the Blues to reimburse for procedures that the medical profession, on balance, agrees should be abandoned. In the search for economies and efficiencies the overt and hidden costs of implementing a new approach need to be considered.

The recent Hatch-Kennedy pressure on the National Institutes of Health to reinstate grants that had been suspended for the development of an artificial heart does not augur well for those who favor placing constraints on high tech. In 1987 the total outlays for biomedical research in the United States exceeded $16.2 billion. About half of the funds were federal appropriations. Any serious slow-down of medical technology would require radical alterations in the nation's research posture, medical education, the specialization of the medical profession, the reorganization of the modern hospitals, a resizing of the pharmaceutical and medical equipment industries, and other institutional changes of incalculable import and impact. Most important, it would require a basic change in the values, attitudes, and behavior of the American people that would lead them to favor stoicism and a shorter life over their present preference for an extended life-span under conditions that yield most of them reasonable satisfaction and freedom from pain.

Epidemiologists have been insisting for a long time that the key to a longer, healthier life owes relatively little to the advances of high-tech medicine. But they have seldom if ever argued that high tech is dysfunctional in pursuing this goal. Small wonder that the American people have voted and will continue to vote with their pocketbooks for more rather than less high-tech medicine, aware as they must be that its prestige exceeds its accomplishments. But that is not unique to high-tech medicine. We seek to strengthen the institutions that have proved themselves, even if partially.

Much has been made of the fact that both the United Kingdom and Canada operate health care systems that are considerably less costly than ours, yet their mortality and morbidity figures are not too different. In this view much of our "excess" outlay, a function of our romance with high tech, is an extravagance, not a necessity. Even if one were to accept this verdict, which has not been proved, the correlative finding is more relevant. Both the United Kingdom and Canada control by legislative action the total funds flowing into the health care system. The presumption that the United States could or should be able to moderate its health care expenditures following the model of these two countries contemplates a great change in the financing of U.S. health care, a change that would place a ceiling on the annual flow of resources into the health care sector. It is possible that at some future date the U.S. will face financing pressures that would encourage or force it to move in that direction. But one will need more than pressures to put a system in place that will effectively control the level of annual funding in a country such as the United States with its scale, scope, and an annual GNP close to $5 trillion. In the absence of such a radical, new system, high-tech medicine appears to have an attractive future.

· II ·

Important
Subsystems

6

Academic Health Centers

A paradox looms on the health care horizon. Here and abroad it is agreed that American medicine has attained its position of world preeminence through the achievements of the academic health center. Yet increasingly the warning is raised that in our zeal to constrain the outlays for health care, we will erode the financial base which has enabled the AHCs to flourish.

There is no singular definition of the characteristics of an AHC and therefore no agreement on the number of institutions that are properly designated as AHCs. For the purpose of this analysis I have identified the forty or so major institutions that comprise, in addition to a medical school, at least one other health professional school (dentistry, nursing, veterinary medicine, and allied health) and that collectively received about 75 percent of the external grants and contracts for biomedical research awarded by the National Institutes of Health (NIH). These research funds amounted in 1984 to approximately $1.2 billion.

The leading AHCs perform several distinct functions: they run a medical school and at least one other health professional school; they conduct a broad spectrum of residency programs and provide advanced training for a large number of fellows; and they perform a considerable volume of basic research and clinical research in the medical school, the principal teaching hospital, and other affiliated hospitals.

Their third mission, in addition to education and research, is caring for patients, particularly inpatients but also outpatients, in their principal affiliate. Many provide professional services for patients in public hospitals as well.

From time to time, some of the AHCs have undertaken demonstration projects aimed at improving the delivery of health care services to designated population groups and have organized and run health maintenance organizations. But up till now such nontraditional efforts in health care delivery have been the exception rather than the rule. Each leg of the metaphoric three-legged stool that describes the functional triad of an AHC—education, research, and patient care—is said to be strengthened by, and dependent upon, its interaction with the other two.

There is a growing unease among the medical leadership that this unique American institution, largely the creation of the post-World War II decades, may be at risk. Supporters of the AHCs have called attention to a number of early warning signs: (1) the leveling off of federal support in real dollars for biomedical research; (2) the elimination of most federal support for medical and other health professional education; (3) the Medi-Cal reforms in 1983 which eliminated on the basis of competitive bidding certain AHCs from serving as authorized providers for Medicaid patients; (4) the entrance of various AHCs into contractual relations with for-profit hospital chains for the purchase, management, or joint operation of their major teaching affiliate in an effort to strengthen access to capital and to improve their revenue position; (5) the year-long moratorium imposed in 1983 by the state of New York on all capital expenditures including several large projects of the principal AHCs in New York City for which approval was pending; (6) the development of preferred-provider organizations, some of which explicitly discriminate against higher-cost AHC hospitals; (7) selected state cutbacks in budgetary support for undergraduate and graduate medical education (GME); and (8) diverse regulatory changes by various states that restrict the freedom of Medicaid patients to select their own providers with an aim of directing these patients to low-cost facilities.[1]

These developments fade into insignificance when placed alongside a number of changes that have been close to the top of the health policy agenda in Washington. These include the recommendation of the Advisory Council for Social Security that Medicare stop reimbursing for GME by 1986; the congressional directive to the Secretary of the Department of Health and Human Services to develop alternatives to the currently in force "pass through" of educational costs under DRGs for teaching hospitals; and early action by Congress to strengthen the Medicare Trust Fund, which will include efforts to reduce inpatient use and total outlays.[2]

Although changes in Medicare are bound to have the greatest immediate impact on the financial position of the AHCs, employer and union-sponsored insurance plans are also being altered. During the last several years there has been considerable restructuring of benefits aimed at encouraging employees to use less expensive providers, and employers have resorted to financial incentives and penalties to influence employee choices. Such efforts are likely to intensify in an atmosphere in which the federal government sets the pace in the search for cost constraints.[3]

The predicament in which the leading AHCs found themselves in the mid-1980s and the challenges that they will confront tomorrow can best be understood by briefly reviewing the ways in which the era of easy money altered their basic structure and functioning during the third of the century following World War II.

The AHC had its origins at the end of the nineteenth century and the beginnings of the twentieth. A number of medical schools, primarily on the East Coast—Harvard, Yale, Columbia, University of Pennsylvania, Johns Hopkins—were then the nation's leaders in medical education, research, and patient care. Medical education centered on undergraduates; research was a minor undertaking financed mostly by modest grants from foundations and performed on a part-time basis by busy clinicians, and even the most sophisticated patient care was severely constrained by what medical knowledge and technique could deliver.

The immediate post-World War II years saw the onset of revolutionary changes on each of these fronts. They can be captured most concisely by reformulating the law of the distinguished business historian, Alfred Chandler, "structure follows function," to read "structure follows finances."[4] It is important to note how new sources of funding affected the mission, organization, and values of the AHCs.

As part of their modernization program for the medical system of the Veterans Administration in 1945–46, Generals Omar Bradley and Paul Hawley sought and obtained the cooperation of the deans of the medical schools who, responding to the new source of financing for residency training, agreed to provide professional services for the VA hospitals.

In 1950 the nation's total expenditure for medical research amounted to only $160 million, with foundations still a significant contributor.[5] But shortly thereafter, the reorganized and expanded National Institutes of Health became the major conduit for new funding for biomedical research, and most of their grants went to the medical schools that were beginning to be transformed into AHCs. Since medical school finances were severely restricted, the ability of the deans to funnel reimbursement for the indirect costs of research into their educational programs proved helpful. This enabled them to expand the number of full-time faculty and to reduce their reliance on volunteer staff.[6]

The rapid extension of hospital insurance with its charge or cost reimbursement for patient care services introduced an important new flow of funds into the major teaching hospitals. The willingness of third-party payers to reimburse for the direct and indirect costs of expanding residency and fellowship programs provided the financial wherewithal to support the restructuring of medical education, which lengthened the physician's period of preparation from five to eight or ten years or more.[7] Although reimbursement for patient services was the major source of new dollars for GME, the NIH also made important contributions through training grants, fellowships, and career development awards.

In the immediate post–World War II years the states were slow to expand their role in financing medical education, but by the mid-1950s several had taken the plunge and more followed, with the result that a large new stream of money for both capital and operating purposes became available. This included state support for the construction of teaching hospitals and for new and expanded facilities for medical research.[8]

In 1963 the federal government moved to allocate substantial sums directly to medical schools, initially for construction and later for operating needs. The effort reached its zenith with the health manpower training legislation of 1971 which authorized capitation for medical and other health professions students.

These multiple streams of new money from the VA, the NIH, insurance, the states, and direct support for medical schools from the federal government were augmented by the passage of Medicare and Medicaid in 1965. By providing liberal reimbursement for inpatient and, to a lesser degree, ambulatory care for the elderly and the poor, they were a source of additional funding for the support of residents and the physicians who supervised their training. Since many AHCs, especially those located in the inner city, had long offered a considerable amount of free and below cost care to the elderly and the poor, the fact that henceforth these patients would no longer be a financial drain but rather a financial asset significantly improved their financial position. For many AHCs money no longer was a scarce resource; space yes, but not money.[9]

The Concomitants of Affluence

A number of major transformations accompanied the cascade of funds into the leading AHCs. The AHC was almost totally removed from university control once it became a contributor to central budgeting rather than its beneficiary. The system of external financing for research reduced the authority of the dean to a point where he was beholden to his principal investigators rather than they to him. The heads of the major departments of the medical school, who in most instances were also the directors of the corresponding services in the principal teaching affiliate, became all-powerful barons by virtue of their control over research funding, residency slots, fellowships, training funds, and hospital beds. Each had his own domain. Prestige and future careers were determined by the esteem of colleagues in the United States and abroad. In addition, the NIH reliance on peer review for grant determination transformed the principal investigator from a professor with collegial values and institutional allegiance into an academic entrepreneur who was in a position to bargain with different schools and often went with the highest bidder.

There was an explosive growth in the number of full-time faculty during the period of expanded funding (1950–1975).[10] Deans and departmental chairmen recognized that if able investigators were recruited to the staff, they could finance them-

selves and also make a contribution to the budget of the department, the medical school, and even the university. This faculty
expansion occurred in both the basic sciences and the clinical
departments. In many institutions, top administrators of the
university and of the medical school were willing to offer tenured appointments on "soft money," that is, to professors who
financed themselves with grant support.

The critical role of research and research funding in the new
value structure of professors profoundly affected their function
as educators. Teaching responsibilities, surely at the undergraduate level, were regarded as secondary to more important activities. *Physicians of the Twenty-First Century*, the recently released report of the Association of American Medical Colleges
Panel on the General Professional Education of the Physician,
chaired by Steven Muller, president of the Johns Hopkins University, is a serious indictment of the neglect of their educational
mission by the medical schools.[11] It is only a slight exaggeration
to state that the single significant innovation in undergraduate
medical education dates from the mid-1950s, when Case Western Reserve set about restructuring its curriculum.

The evolution of GME was even stranger. It came under the
professional dominance of the several specialty societies and the
residency review committees, with the teaching hospital playing
a significant role as financier and employer of residents. Not to
overstate the case, it should be noted that the senior medical
school professors, in their roles as directors of hospital departments, were important participants. The expanded spectrum of
residency programs in the largest AHCs, frequently more than
twenty, and the concomitant growth in the total number of
residents, in some cases as many as 1,000, brought with it important consequences for hospital operations, financing, and patient care.[12]

Regarding residency training, the dominant view is that its
proliferation was broadly beneficial: the presence of residents
provided the hospital with full-time house staff, raised the level
of clinical acumen by having novitiates challenge their elders,
and encouraged a more "scientific" approach to both diagnosis
and therapy. The negatives are usually ignored or minimized:
unnecessary testing and procedures, extended patient stays, increased hospital expenditures.

The universality of residency training for graduates of U.S. medical schools as well as expanded opportunities for many foreign medical school graduates to receive similar training had significant effects for the treatment of poor and indigent patients in public hospitals. This occurred initially in the VA hospitals and later in many municipal, county, and state hospitals that looked to the AHCs for professional support. Before World War II, many of these hospitals depended on salaried staff supplemented by volunteer physicians, but in more recent decades most patient care services have been provided by residents under the supervision of attending specialists.[13]

In the decades of new, increased funding for the AHCs, there was relatively little pressure on university, medical school, or hospital trustees to consider joint planning and improved governance. The several bodies had enough to do just to stay on top of their respective responsibilities. The ever larger flow of funds enabled each of the key administrative officials to set and maintain a fast pace on a steeply graded trajectory. If one or another source of anticipated funding fell through, there was always another to draw on. As businessmen know so well, a sustained period of expansion is the best short-term device for papering over difficult problems.[14]

Challenge and Response

The high point in the financing of the AHCs came in the early 1970s. Even though NIH funding had leveled off, Medicare and Medicaid reimbursement plus direct federal support for medical education and teaching hospitals' recourse to the private capital markets for construction funds kept the money sluices open. The reduction and subsequent elimination of federal support for medical education in the late 1970s was the first serious setback in the absence of any alternative funding source. That lack, however, was not altogether intractable. Many AHCs, especially those under private auspices, decided to raise medical school tuition and to establish or expand physician practice plans, which produced revenue to cover the salaries of many of the full-time staff and contributed to departmental and medical school budgets.

Almost without notice, practice plan income has within the

last decade come to represent the single largest source of funding available to private medical schools (about one-third), amounting at the extreme to $50 or $60 million a year. The typical situation finds a large medical school with a great many different plans, each departmentally based and operated, with considerable hassle as to the amounts that are skimmed off to support the less affluent basic science departments.

A few of the most distinguished AHCs have been able to attract large sums from major domestic or foreign corporations to undertake research in designated areas. The contractual arrangements vary, but most donors are given the first opportunity to exploit findings that may result in proprietary products.[15]

Although the years from the mid-seventies to the mid-eighties have not been easy for the AHCs, they have all come through, some in better, some in worse condition. But the next decade— 1985–1995—will really put them to the test. The conventional wisdom is that third-party payers will recognize that the costs of medical education must be covered in one fashion or another; that the major teaching hospitals need a reimbursement system which reflects the higher intensity of care that they provide for many patients; that the care of the indigent must be paid for; and that the nation must continue to support biomedical research at an appropriate level. Under such conditions the AHCs should be able to survive without serious scarring. For the reasons that are elaborated below, I believe that such an assessment is unduly optimistic and the AHCs are much more vulnerable than is assumed.

Medical education. One of the potent factors contributing to the heavy flow of funds into AHCs in the 1950–1975 period was the widespread belief that the country needed more and better trained physicians. Today the dominant view is quite different. More often we hear that the nation may face an oversupply of physicians and that excessive numbers of specialists and subspecialists swell the total cost of the health care system.[16] Duke University and the University of Pennsylvania have indicated that they will cut back on their undergraduate enrollments, and the political leadership in several Midwestern states is discussing a staged cutback of 20 percent over the next few years in their schools. The shift in the national mood is best exemplified by the fact that the AHCs, which originally resisted pressures by the states and the federal government to expand their medical school capacity, are now blamed for the oversupply of physicians.

There are also stirrings on the GME front. An increasing number of specialty societies have been taking another look at their numbers and several residency review committees have increased their requirements with an aim of improving quality, a move antecedent to reducing their future membership.[17] It is difficult to forecast in the mid-1980s, five years after publication of the Graduate Medical Education National Advisory Committee report, whether and how quickly the new atmosphere will lead to actions that will effect significant reductions in undergraduate and graduate medical education. As yet, there is no consensus—and none may emerge—about desirable or necessary measures.[18]

At the same time, the odds are strong that third-party payers will seek to eliminate the cost of GME from reimbursement for patient care services. In the process of developing alternative financing, the scale and length of residency and fellowship support will be reduced, probably not to one year, the drastic suggestion of the Inspector General of Health and Human Services (HHS), but more likely to three years, as proposed by Robert Petersdorf of the University of California (San Diego).[19]

The AHCs may also find that the federal government will seek to cut back on residency support in the hospitals of the Veterans Administration and that some of their other public hospital affiliates may decide to rely less on residents and more on salaried staff to treat their patients now that the easing of the physician supply facilitates their recruitment.

As states examine ways to control their health care outlays, they may follow an early lead by California, which reduced (modestly) its budgeted residency slots on the ground that the state had no need to increase its future supply of physicians. A New York gubernatorial commission has recently reviewed the scale and scope of residency training within the state's jurisdiction. New York City, which has approximately 2.5 percent of the nation's population, trains about 12 percent of the nation's residents, many of whom relocate to other states to practice.

Medical research. During the period of liberal financing for biomedical research, many of the AHCs vastly increased their medical school faculty both in the basic sciences and in the clinical departments. When the research dollars, in real terms, began to level off and some of the researchers were no longer able to attract new grants to cover their salaries and expenses, many of them were shifted to the hospital budget or were subsidized from practice plan revenues. The outlook for the continuance of hospital support is jeopardized by the shift to DRGs, and it is becoming increasingly clear that a medical school that relies heavily on practice plan income will soon find that many of its faculty are so busy practicing that they have little time for research and less for students. Paradoxically, such a medical school will, after a detour of several decades, return close to its starting point, when it relied primarily on volunteer physicians for clinical teaching.

Possibly the most serious consequence of the radical shift from a period of easy money to an increasingly constrained budgetary environment is the reduced scope of many AHCs to provide opportunities for young researchers to gain a foothold on the academic ladder that would enable the more talented to attain a tenured position later. Since they have a large complement of tenured faculty with an average age of less than fifty, few AHCs are able to make more than an occasional tenured track appointment. Nothing is more threatening to the continuing vitality of the AHCs than their present and prospective faculty resources, with large numbers past their productive peak and limited opportunities to appoint younger men and women.[20]

The major teaching hospital. As noted earlier, the teaching hospital played a critical role in helping the AHC achieve its position of prominence. It was the site where the AHC demonstrated its capacity to deliver the best of inpatient care. With its large number of residents and fellows it became an important educational resource, perhaps more important than the medical school itself, which concentrated on undergraduates. As the "cash cow," the teaching hospital was in a good position to make the heavy investments required to keep the AHC at the cutting edge of diagnosis and therapy, and, as we have seen, it also contributed to the salaries of many of the AHCs teaching and research staff.

For several reasons the teaching hospital may no longer be able to maintain this supportive role, the most important being the changed reimbursement climate, the shift away from inpatient care, and the need for organizational initiatives to protect and enlarge its market share.

Let us briefly inspect each in turn. The DRG system will surely not be the last word in hospital reimbursement, but it speaks to the sea change that has occurred. Third-party payers are determined to moderate their outlays for hospital care and to avoid having to pay providers whatever they demand. The large teaching hospitals will almost surely convince third-party payers that they are entitled to a higher reimbursement rate because of the intensity of treatment that they provide. But this adjustment will be far short of the much higher reimbursement rate that they have long received for all their patients. Moreover, hospitals will no longer be free to cross-subsidize, surely not to the same extent as in the past, when they loaded the costs that were not covered onto paying and insured patients. The odds are strong, even overwhelming, that the major teaching hospitals will not continue to enjoy the substantial differential in reimbursement rates that has prevailed between them and community hospitals over the past several decades. They will be under increasing pressure to become price-competitive.

Some time must pass before we can be sure, but the trends suggest that the United States has passed the peak in days of hospitalization and that the future, despite a larger and older population, will see a decline, possibly even a steep decline. Numerous explanations are given: the pressures that the DRGs are exerting on hospitals and physicians to reduce length of stay; the recent growth of HMOs, whose members have a much lower rate of hospital admission; the shift to ambulatory treatment facilities (surgi-center, physicians' offices, and other sites); monetary and other incentives that employers are using to discourage unnecessary hospitalization; and, most important, technological advances that underlie many of the above. Improvements in imaging and in anesthesiology surely have contributed greatly to the recent trend toward ambulatory surgery, which is still far from leveling off.[21]

The major teaching hospitals of the AHCs face a further challenge. For many years they were recognized and sought out by the well-off patients in search of superior medical treatment. In the intervening decades many of the affluent moved to the suburbs and many of the young specialists whom the AHCs had trained established a practice there. In the presence of good hospital and staff support, these suburban specialists found that only rarely did they have to refer a patient to the AHC. Most patients could be treated effectively in their community hospital. The combination of these two trends—reduced hospital days and fewer referrals—is likely over time to leave many large teaching hospitals with surplus beds.

If the foregoing scenario of tightened reimbursement, declining hospital use, and fewer referrals proves correct, the major teaching hospitals will be under increasing pressure to restructure themselves to assure their future. They will need to work out new arrangements with physicians, hospitals, clinics, and prepaid group practices to provide a flow of patients adequate in numbers and clinical mix to fill their beds. That will not be easy to accomplish given the preferences and predilections of the medical school faculty whose aims and goals are only partially congruent with the optimal operation of the hospital. The much touted synergism of the past may turn into a serious encumbrance.

There is little that is upbeat in the foregoing summary overview: a shrinking educational enterprise; declining reimbursement for GME; level financing for medical research; a top-heavy tenured faculty with few openings for younger people; a teaching hospital that faces a declining demand for inpatient care; and a more competitive environment.

But all is not bleak; far from it. The large teaching hospitals in states with waivers are not doing poorly. In a few states that have adopted "all-payer systems" the AHCs are able to continue to treat a considerable number of indigent patients without risking insolvency. In some areas (Boston and New York City) the AHCs continue to attract a large number of patients who will pay a premium for the quality of care that the AHCs are singularly able to provide.

Various AHCs, depending on their circumstances and profit margins, have begun to reposition themselves. Some universities are reorganizing their principal teaching hospitals as separate corporations so that they will be buffered from the uncertainties of the hospital environment. Some teaching hospitals are working out new arrangements with their attending staff. Still others are entering into alliances with potential competitors or developing relationships with HMOs and PPOs which will provide a more certain stream of patients, many of whom will require tertiary care. The innovations are many and diverse, and more are surely developing.[22]

Direction for Restructuring the AHCs

We are now in a better position to suggest a range of possible actions that the AHCs could engage in, individually and collectively, to contribute to the advance of medical knowledge and medical practice in the difficult decade ahead. The challenges that they will face include intensified efforts by government and insurance to slow their outlays for health care; a more competitive environment among health care deliverers with AHCs confronted by price-cutting for the first time; a growing conviction among many sectors of the public that the nation has moved from a shortage to a surplus of physicians with consequent implications for the financing of medical education; and a diffuse uneasiness among the public about many dimensions of the health care system, from the perception of excessive earnings by certain groups of specialists to questions about the utility of high-tech interventions to prolong the lives of patients who have little prospect of regaining functionality.[23]

Clearly, the AHCs might adopt alternative policy approaches to meet these challenges. The following recommendations are grouped under four headings: medical education and research, the delivery of health care, governance, and public opinion. In the interest of brevity, the directions for action that the AHCs might consider are presented without the supporting facts and figures.

Medical education and research. Medical educators should take the initiative and seek to persuade state legislatures and the federal government that it makes sense to cut back moderately on undergraduate enrollments, but only if the inflow of foreign-trained graduates is effectively controlled. Further, if such action is decided upon, it would be preferable for state legislators not to reduce the financing of medical schools, but to merge or close one or more of the weaker schools rather than impose an across-the-board reduction for all schools. In the face of likely reductions in federal funding for student aid, private schools with higher tuition must redouble their efforts to secure additional grant and loan funds so that they do not find themselves in the undesirable position of admitting only applicants from affluent families.

Strategy with respect to faculty should emphasize reduction in total numbers, early retirement of tenured professors, assurance of a reasonable number of tenure-track openings for talented young academicians, and the recognition that there are distinct limits to dependence upon practice-plan income for covering salaries because of inevitable conflicts between the practice time required to produce such income and the time required for teaching and research. Also, despite the many difficulties that confront medical school administrators and faculty, the challenges for educational reform set out in the Muller report need to be addressed.

It is likely that Congress will explore, and probably act on, the recommendation of the Advisory Council on Social Security to alter the basis of payment for the direct (and indirect) costs of graduate medical education.[24] The AHCs should develop one or more proposals that, if adopted, would provide GME with independent funding, proposals that will appeal not only to Congress but also to other third-party payers. Such proposals should recognize that Congress and other third-party payers will not be inclined to earmark such funds.

The principal source of funds for medical research has been the National Institutes of Health. In 1984 Congress increased their appropriation to over $5 billion, approximately $575 million above the administration's recommendation. However, in light of the deepening difficulties facing the federal budget, it is unlikely that the AHCs can anticipate any better than level funding in the years ahead. With major teaching hospitals facing a more uncertain financial future, there will be less opportunity for them to contribute to the support of researchers who fail to obtain external grants. The AHCs face the unpropitious outlook of no significant new sources of funding for medical research.

The most important challenge to the AHCs on the research front is the need to ensure that they have openings for talented young academicians to pursue a research career, and that the best of them have the opportunity to attain a tenure position. A stagnant level of funding makes it difficult, but not impossible, to create a reasonable number of such positions, but only if the AHCs adopt appointment, tenure, and retirement policies consistent with this critical goal.

The delivery of health care. The current provisions requiring Medicare, under its DRG reimbursement system, to take account of the higher intensity of care that AHCs provide for many patients are almost certain to be revised shortly. It is critically important for the AHCs to assure that the new system continues to reflect their higher costs, including those incurred by virtue of their designation as the sole regional providers for selected expensive services, such as treating burn victims and caring for high-risk neonates. The AHCs face the similar task of convincing state governments and insurance carriers that they are entitled to reimbursement for the above-average costs of high intensity care.

AHCs must also seek to convince third-party payers that it would be adverse public policy if they were forced, because of lack of adequate reimbursement, to deny treatment to large numbers of the indigent who have traditionally depended upon them for medical care. Public hospitals are seldom in a position to admit and treat effectively a much enlarged flow of these patients. Several states have implemented "all-payer systems," which seek to distribute the costs of charity care among all hospitals in proportion to their volume of indigent patients. This approach, or variants having the same objective, should be further explored and refined.

PPOs and other innovative financing and delivery systems are being introduced with the aim of controlling health care costs. AHCs must be on the alert to avoid being excluded by the marketers of such plans simply because of their higher costs. As noted earlier, a partial explanation for these costs is the fact that they provide services not available in other hospitals. AHCs must convince state officials that they should be given the opportunity to compete fairly with lower-cost providers.[25]

The principal teaching affiliates of many AHCs will probably face in the near or middle term a significant downscaling of their inpatient capacity as the result of several mutually reinforcing trends: major pressure from DRGs to reduce the average length of stay; an accelerated shift to ambulatory surgery; the growth of HMOs with their much lower frequency of hospital admissions; and fewer referrals because of the redistribution of specialists to the suburbs and beyond.[26]

The prospective reversal of the earlier trend toward the expansion of inpatient care in favor of ambulatory services presents a major challenge to the AHCs whose teaching and clinical research as well as patient care are focused almost exclusively on inpatients. The AHCs are not well positioned to shift their focus, and they face the added challenge that up till now the financing of GME has been predicated on reimbursement for inpatients. Nevertheless, it is unlikely that the AHCs will be able to evade the need to reposition themselves because the trend to ambulatory care will be irresistible.

Governance. We have noted that in the long period of easy money relatively little attention was paid to improving the governance and management of AHCs.[27] Now that money has become much tighter, this characteristically loose governance represents a major problem for many AHCs. Some universities have moved to sell or contract, usually with a for-profit enterprise, for the management of their principal affiliated hospitals in order to protect themselves from the threat of large operating deficits. In other cases, their motivation has been to obtain needed capital for modernization or expansion. If large teaching hospitals should experience serious balance-sheet difficulties in the years ahead—a distinct possibility in light of the decline in patient days and greater price competition—more universities will explore alternatives to their present arrangements.

We noted earlier that in the years of open-handed funding for medical research and GME, power shifted from the deans to departmental chairmen and principal investigators. It will not be easy for medical schools to reverse this trend, but if they are to respond to the many critical needs that have been identified, from reforming the curriculum to implementing constructive personnel policies that will assure a vital faculty, a strengthening of the central medical school administration is essential.

The symbiosis of the medical school and its primary clinical affiliate, which has been a major source of strength during the long era of prosperity, may turn into a hindrance, if not a fatal liability, for the hospital in the years ahead. The hospital must move aggressively to work out a great many new linkages with a variety of providers—to assure itself the numbers and types of patients who can make optimal use of its sophisticated services. It is far from clear that the medical school faculty is the most suitable, much less the only, party to such restructuring. The years ahead will see innovation and possibly quite radical changes in the relations between many medical school faculties and their major teaching affiliates.

Two major incentives for new and, in many instances, looser relations between medical schools and their principal affiliates will be the need of the teaching hospital to protect and improve its referral streams and the medical school faculty's preoccupation with other activities. In the tussle between hospital survival and medical school control, it is likely that the former will move to expand its degrees of freedom to respond to the changing market, and the medical school faculty will probably have to acquiesce.

Public opinion. In a democracy such as ours, public opinion has a critical influence on the actions of decision-makers in the governmental, nonprofit, and profit-seeking arenas. The golden age of the AHCs (1950–1975) owed a great deal to the strong support of the American people for all aspects of the medical enterprise—education, research, and patient care. While public opinion is still broadly supportive of the AHCs, this favorable climate can no longer be taken for granted. The AHCs need to improve their public information efforts to gain and maintain support for their critical missions.

One line to take would be to disabuse the American people, who have been led to believe that there are almost no limits to what modern medicine can accomplish. The AHCs have surely contributed to this view of medical omnipotence, and as a result many citizens expect physicians to be victorious in most encounters with the threat of death. A more realistic set of public expectations about the capacity of modern medicine would protect the AHCs from overreaction to disappointments. Second, total medical research funding, from all sources, amounted in 1984 to something over $10 billion or approximately 2.5 percent of all health care outlays. Although that was a good year for congressional appropriations for medical research, the future may not always be so supportive. The AHCs should make more of an effort to inform the public about the potentialities and limitations of medical research in the short, medium, and long run. Exaggerated claims, such as winning the war on cancer, must be avoided. But reasonable claims that justify enlarged funding should be presented in a way that would commend them to a mature electorate.

The medical leadership of the AHCs also has a responsibility to help the public understand the links between medicine and health, between providers and consumers, and to point out the obligation of the individual citizen to protect and maintain his or her health. Admittedly, these educational challenges are often viewed as diversionary by busy academicians and researchers, but they must recognize that no profession and no institution can look to a secure future without the support of an informed, understanding public. That is the lesson of the past and the injunction for the future.

A Concluding Note

Conventional wisdom views the AHC as a modern, uniquely American institution, and so it is. But it would be a mistake to conclude that its uniqueness assures its continuing survival and vitality. Half a century ago in a short essay on "The Decline of Antiquity" I noted that the decline of the civilizations of Greece and later of Rome resulted from the fact that both the Athenian and the Roman military governments were ultimately unable to extract from the conquered nations the resources needed for the support of its top-heavy superstructure.[28]

As I discuss it at length in a book written with George Vojta,[29] in periods of rapid and prolonged expansion the large corporation accumulates a "cushion." Growth, however, simultaneously produces a more complex organizational structure and a decision-making mechanism that is slow to react. As a consequence, highly successful corporations find it increasingly difficult to respond to complex changes in their environment, and thus lose their edge and initiative and begin to decline.

The AHC is similarly characterized by a complex structure and a slowly responding decision mechanism. In the changing environment ahead its future appears troubled because of uncertainty that it will be able to use its resources, human and physical, in new ways to assure continuing productivity in an era of constrained funding.

At a conference in the spring of 1987,[30] the deans and hospital directors of five prestigious AHCs on the East Coast, in the Midwest, and the West did not report unfavorably on their current and prospective status. Quite the contrary: their institutions showed a strong bottom line, and they did not discern any serious threats on the horizon. These major teaching hospitals had responded to a lower level of inpatient utilization through a series of adjustments that included some downsizing, a reduction in personnel, more aggressive outreach for referrals, arrangements with managed care systems to ensure additional inpatient admissions, expanded ambulatory care services, provision of new high-tech programs, and still other managerial and marketing innovations.

Such actions enabled them to adapt satisfactorily to the introduction of DRGs and to the modest reductions in Medicare support for GME. No reference was made to the fact that the original base for the DRGs had been miscalculated, resulting in unduly high payments to hospitals or to the excessively liberal factor for "extraordinary" expenses incurred by the AHCs by virtue of their teaching mission and their disproportionate number of complicated, critically ill patients.

So much for the hospital side of the AHCs. The academic representatives were less sanguine. The shift of patients from inpatient to ambulatory care settings made it more difficult for them to provide properly supervised clinical training to both undergraduates and house staff. Moreover, same-day surgery and the pressure for early discharge meant that residents had progressively less, if any, opportunity to see the individual patient before, during, and after an acute illness, and were thereby deprived of an essential learning experience.

It was becoming increasingly difficult, in the views of the department chairs, to obtain requisite funding for clinical research—funding that, in less pressured days, the hospital had been able to provide, at least in part. True, by increasing the volume of ambulatory consultations the funding for clinical research could be increased, but this was not cost-free. The preoccupation of the full-time staff with diagnosing and treating patients had encroached on the time available for teaching students and residents.

Other disturbing trends were the new conflicts of interest that resulted when faculty members had an equity stake in various delivery systems, the difficulties of developing an adequate number of ambulatory care sites for teaching purposes, and the impact of straitened university budgets on faculty staffing.

In sum, the directors of the major teaching hospitals reported that after a period of some turbulence and uncertainty, they had been able to steer their institutions into calmer waters and were reasonably confident about the future. Although the deans and department chairs were less optimistic, the difficulties that they noted were not of an order to pose a major threat to their educational and research missions. There is no reason to question these reports of the recent experience of the major AHCs and their favorable position, both financial and educational, in 1987.

Yet I differ radically in my assessment of what the future holds for these leading institutions, long on the cutting edge of the US medical care system. A number of important factors that were either overlooked or underestimated by the conferees suggest that they may have been unjustifiably optimistic about the future.

(1) At the time it had only been three years since the institution of the new DRG system, and this period was characterized by a large amount of slack in the hospital system that grew out of seventeen years of cost or charge reimbursement. Ratcheting down from a position of long-term surplus is not the same as being forced to confront a long-term environment of fiscal constraint.

(2) The operation of the DRG system is flawed in that it is predicated on a base that has favored the vendors; while Congress may not take action to lower the base, the most recent budget reconciliation proposal would increase the level of hospital payment for the next fiscal year only from 1 percent to 2 percent.[31] With the inflation of hospital and health care costs in the double-digit range, the belated correction of the DRG base by restraining the annual adjustment factor will lead to widespread anguish.

(3) The probable continuing declines in inpatient utilization will increase the pressure on the larger AHCs to downscale further and inevitably elicit additional tensions.

(4) The growing "surplus" of physicians, in the aggregate and particularly in the specialties and subspecialties, that reflects

the expanded capacity of medical schools and residency training programs, has serious financial implications. Congress will very likely authorize, in the near future, continuing reductions in funding for GME and the related costs of teaching hospitals.

(5) Large reductions in Medicare expenditures are recommended in the president's budget for 1990. The Congressional Budget Office's analysis of the budget for 1990 and the years beyond also contains sizable alternative reductions for Medicare.[32]

(6) Decreasing inpatient utilization has serious import for the need for teaching sites in ambulatory care settings; yet, at the present time, financing arrangements for the latter are largely nonexistent.

(7) There is evidence of growing discontent among medical school students and residents with many aspects of their educational and training experience. However, these serious criticisms have elicited little response from AHCs. If the training of the next generation of the nation's physicians remains the principal task of the AHCs, this diffuse student discontent should be a major area of concern over and above questions of future financing.

(8) Finally, we are six years into an expansion of the U.S. economy, and this brings the next recession that much closer. A recession that led to or was precipitated by an international financial and trade crisis could result in major readjustments in the U.S. public and private economy, with serious adverse effects on the health care sector and AHCs.

If the AHC leadership proves as successful in lobbying Congress and the public in the future as it has in the past, the dangers identified above—and adverse actions by state legislatures and employers—might be forestalled or minimized. But such an outcome appears to be increasingly problematic in the face of the growing excess of hospital beds and physicians, the growth of managed care delivery systems, and large-scale increases of total health care outlays that, at the end of 1987, reached $500 billion or 11.2% of the gross national product—both new highs.

If I were the dean of a medical school or the director of a large teaching affiliate, I would be operating on the assumption that the recent past provides few clues to the future. The major AHCs will survive but not without undergoing major trauma.

7

Foundations and the Nation's Health Agenda

Philanthropic foundations and the U.S. health care system have had a dynamic and varied relationship. This chapter presents an overview of these relations from the beginning of the century, then looks ahead to the challenge that foundations will confront in determining the optimal investment of their health care dollars as the century draws to a close. The intent of the analysis is to identify and assess basic issues rather than to seek definitive judgments.

The Long View

Revisionist historians have questioned whether the reform of medical education after 1910 should be attributed exclusively to the Carnegie Foundation and Abraham Flexner, given the long preparatory efforts of the American Medical Association. Nonetheless, the foundation and Flexner do deserve most of the recognition that has usually been accorded them for their leadership.

Early patrons of biomedical research. In the field of biomedical research, the Rockefeller Foundation and the Rockefeller Institute are the acknowledged founding patrons, having established the Rockefeller Institute for Medical Research and supported efforts of the leading medical schools to advance basic and clinical research via the modernization of the medical school curriculum. The Rockefeller Foundation also played a leading role in the public health arena through its support of research in parasitic diseases and of large-scale efforts to translate promising research findings into action programs. Under the direction of Alan Gregg, its long-time vice-president for medical affairs, the Rockefeller Foundation also took the initiative in the 1930s to strengthen the teaching of psychiatry in a number of leading medical schools by offering long-term financial support and guidance.

In 1940, just prior to the U.S. entering the war, foundations accounted for $12 million of annual grants for biomedical research out of a national expenditure of $45 million, or almost 30 percent of the total. The expenditures of the federal government for biomedical research in that year amounted to just $3 million, a proportion which underscores the significant role that foundations played in the early financing of research.

Improving the U.S. medical system. In the prewar era the major foundations with interests in health contributed significantly to strengthening medical schools, biomedical research, and public health programs. They sought to elevate the level of U.S. medicine to equal the best in Western Europe. They also tried, through their support of the Committee on the Costs of Medical Care, to achieve a new national consensus about how the delivery of health care could be made more effective and more equitable. The effort failed, in part because the Great Depression intervened. In 1932, however, the commission produced the most intensive analysis of the U.S. health care system that had yet been developed; its quality has not been matched in the succeeding half century.

The best testimonial to the role of foundations up to World War II is found in the recommendations of the Medical Advisory Committee to Vannevar Bush, included in his 1945 report to President Truman, *Science: the Endless Frontier.* The advisory committee recommended that the federal government enlarge its support for biomedical research, emphasizing, however, that government should not become the sole source of financial support. Rather, the advisory committee noted, it was important to maintain an environment in which researchers could look to alternative sources of support, in particular foundations. The extent to which World War II was a watershed in the structure and magnitude of the biomedical research enterprise is suggested by this comparison: in 1945 it was the considered opinion of the advisory committee that a reasonable starting level of federal support for biomedical research would be around $5 million a year. Forty years later, in 1986, total federal outlays amounted to $7.2 billion, 240 times as great after correcting for inflation.

The Post-World War II Era

A schematic reconstruction of the four decades since World War II would divide these years into two periods. The first, from 1945 to 1972, witnessed the rapid expansion of the U.S. health care system. In the subsequent fifteen years efforts at cost containment and the introduction of more efficient and economical systems of delivering care have commanded center stage.

Rapid growth of the health care sector. In the earlier decades all sectors underwent explosive growth, some earlier, some later. This dynamism was reflected in the building and enlargement of hospitals; the cascade of federal funds for biomedical research; state initiatives leading to the establishment of new medical schools; the growth of private insurance; the passage of Medicare and Medicaid; federal actions to increase the physician supply by expanding our medical education plant and by facilitating the immigration of physicians trained abroad; and federal and state support to enlarge the supply of nurses and allied health personnel. Only one sector lost out: it was the area commonly subsumed under the rubric of public health, which includes such diverse activities as health education, school health services, the control of environmental hazards, and other facets of health promotion and disease prevention.

The years 1945 to 1972 proved to be the most dynamic period in the history of American medicine, yet the major foundations had only a marginal impact on the dramatic developments that transpired. They contributed to the construction and equipment of hospitals and academic health centers; they continued to support biomedical research and the training of research personnel, although their dollars were dwarfed by those appropriated by the Congress; occasionally they endowed a professorship at an established or new medical school, and they made modest funds available to selected teaching hospitals that sought to strengthen their research and training activities. A few foundations attempted to encourage the recruitment of specific groups of health personnel via programs to assist minorities wishing to enter medicine; others attempted to strengthen nurse leadership by supporting education at the masters' and doctoral levels.

In 1950 total health care expenditures amounted to $13.5 billion or 4.7 percent of GNP; the comparable figures for 1972 were $94 billion or 7.7 percent of GNP. The GNP had expanded more than fourfold (in current dollars) and the contribution of health care outlays as a percentage of the much enlarged GNP base had increased by just under two-thirds. The cumulative weight of the new flows of funding by private insurance, federal, state, and local government appropriations and out-of-pocket payments by consumers swamped the donations of philanthropy and overwhelmed the contributions of foundations to the health care sector.

Throughout this tumultuous period of rapid expansion and change, foundations took relatively little initiative to study and evaluate any of the high priority issues in the interest of informing public policy. They were not among the principal advocates for passage of the Hill-Burton Act; neither did they warn against the dangers of constructing a large number of small hospitals in outlying areas that could not recruit and retain competent staffs. They provided at best limited guidance to the public about future physician supply until 1970, when the Carnegie Commission on Higher Education presented its report strongly recommending accelerated expansion of medical education. This was just six years before Congress concluded that the physician shortage was over.

The revision of the immigration statutes in 1965 facilitated the entry into the United States of foreign-trained physicians who were encouraged to become licensed, acquire citizenship, and practice medicine. No foundation or group of foundations interested in health care took the initiative to assess the implications and the wisdom of this national policy. There was no major foundation effort to evaluate the transformation of U.S. medical education from a system focused on the preparation of general practitioners to one that emphasized the training of specialists and subspecialists. Neither did the foundations examine the implications of this change for the public's ability to have ready access to primary care and for the long-term costs of a medical system increasingly dependent on specialization.

Perhaps more surprising is that foundations were not in the

forefront of efforts to broaden access to health care for the elderly and the poor even though the states and the federal government had begun to wrestle with the issue in the 1950s. In the final legislative struggle in the early 1960s preceding the passage of Medicare and Medicaid, the principal contestants were the Congress and the AMA. No foundation had probed the issues in depth or had produced a study that pointed to alternative resolutions.

In sum, while American medicine was radically transformed in the 1945–1972 era, it is hard to identify the leverage that any foundation exercised on any of these major developments. Foundations continued to use their funds constructively on several discrete fronts, but by no stretch of the imagination were they among the movers and shakers. They had been displaced by health care lobbyists, the chairmen of key committees in the Senate and the House, and by senior personnel in the National Institutes of Health. At the helm were those who had leading roles in determining the amount of federal funds that would be made available for health and those who could influence the allocation of these funds.

The past two decades. By the early 1970s the long period of expansion of the health care system and the growing euphoria that accompanied it were running out. In 1970 President Nixon proclaimed that the nation faced a health care crisis because of steeply rising costs. In 1972 Congress legislated the establishment of professional standards review organizations with the aim of slowing the steep rise in Medicare outlays. Both the President and the Congress looked favorably on federal assistance to health maintenance organizations in the expectation that their expansion would help moderate total health care expenditures. In 1976 it seemed that national health insurance—off the nation's health agenda since the late 1940s—might reappear, but it was swept aside by the unremitting upward trend in health care expenditures.

Betty L. Dooley has surveyed the role of foundation giving in health care in the much more contained economic environment of 1975–1983.[1] If money is a measure of power and influence, the $712 million total of grants earmarked for health by foundations in 1983 must be seen in the context of an annual national outlay for health care of $355 billions. Foundation grants accounted for just 0.2 percent.

A closer look, however, reveals that in two areas—health professional education training and health services research—foundation funding played a much more important role. Foundations had concluded that, given their limited funds, they could not make much impact on the actual provision of patient care or even on the funding of biomedical research. But they did have an opportunity to capture some high ground by supporting experimental and demonstration programs aimed at developing new models for delivering care and by financing projects in health services research whose results promised to point directions for making the system more efficient and equitable.

In contrast to the foundation's minimal contribution to total health care outlays, their dollars paced federal expenditures for the training of physicians (a ratio of five federal dollars to every one dollar for foundations) and of nurses (a ratio of three federal dollars to one foundation dollar). The area in which foundation dollars were relatively most prominent was health services research, to which foundations contributed about two-thirds as much as the federal government.

The nation's health agenda. It may be helpful to recall some of the major issues that found their way onto the nation's health agenda during the last fifteen years of increasing public preoccupation with cost containment: (1) improving the efficacy of health care delivery systems; (2) increasing the output of primary care physicians; (3) curbing the institutionalization of many acute and chronic care patients and treating them in alternative sites; (4) responding to the needs of the rapidly increasing numbers of the elderly; (5) concern for the increasing numbers of the poor and the near-poor not covered by insurance or Medicaid; (6) the potential and the limits of the competitive market's ability to allocate health resources and services; (7) the growing importance of life-style changes in health maintenance; (8) developing national policy to respond to the Graduate Medical Education National Advisory Committee (GMENAC) report of impending physician surplus; (9) medical malpractice; (10) quality control measures; and (11) finding answers to periodic nurse shortages.

Participation of foundations. Unquestionably some foundations made serious attempts to address one or more of these issues; a few of the larger foundations mounted efforts to meet some of them. But again, with the advantage of hindsight, what does a trial balance sheet show? A number of foundations helped to design new forms of service delivery aimed at achieving some moderation in the costs of care. Others took the initiative to support residency training for family care practitioners, although it is difficult to identify a major evaluation effort that attempted to assess the potential and limits of the future role of family practitioners. More significant is the fact that, after a thirty year period that had emphasized the training of specialists and subspecialists, no foundation explored the possible gains to the American people from a reduction in specialty training.

Further, the dominance of the hospital in the health care system went largely uncriticized. This is not to deny that more than one foundation supported demonstration projects aimed at improving ambulatory care services to middle class or poor patients. However, no foundation looked hard at the dominance and the centrality of the hospital in the health care delivery system despite the hospitals' growing consumption of total health care dollars.

Several foundations funded projects directed at improving medical services to the elderly, but many aspects of caring for them remain unexamined or superficially examined. For instance, the potential of private insurance to cover catastrophic long-term care had been largely neglected. Estimates of the current needs for additional nursing home capacity for the years 2000 and 2010 differ widely. But there is no clarity about the areas in which home care is to be preferred over institutional care for the incapacitated and the frail elderly.

Several foundations are exploring alternative approaches to providing coverage for the 35 to 40 million Americans who currently lack health insurance. This number, parenthetically, is likely to increase as the proportion of the work force that is employed less than full-time/full-year grows and as more workers are employed in small enterprises. This issue, critical as it is, is only one manifestation of the uncertain durability and viability of our present highly pluralistic approach to paying for health care. As noted earlier, national health insurance almost made it back onto the nation's health agenda in the mid-1970s. It is likely to reemerge during the coming decade.

But the unanticipated expansion of for-profit hospitals and for-profit health delivery chains and the more recent declines in their profitability and long-term prospects were largely ignored by foundations, although one might have expected them to adopt a protective position toward the nonprofit sector. Moreover, the growing governmental support for competition as the preferred mechanism to restrain costs and improve the delivery of services—a challenge to the principles that have guided the U.S. health care system since the beginning of this century and before—should have been examined in depth and the conclusions widely debated. No foundation, however, took the lead to inform and instruct the public.

Only a few off-beat individuals and institutions have challenged the unremitting pursuit of therapeutics to the substantial neglect of prevention and rehabilitation that has until recently characterized the U.S. health care system. Even the foundations with a history of achievement in the arena of public health did not explore the possible benefits of redirecting resources away from therapeutics to prevention for the nation's health and for its pocketbook.

Despite their long-term interest and involvement in health professional education and training, the foundations did not sponsor an in-depth assessment of the findings and recommendations of the GMENAC report, which put in play the future supply of physicians and also the supply of and demand for most other types of health professionals. Seven years after GMENAC, the AMA House of Delegates finally adopted the official position that GMENAC predictions of surplus by the end of the century were valid and that new policy initiatives were required to reduce the future flows into the profession.

When one recalls the modest share of total health care spending that their grants cover, it should come as no surprise that foundations have been at best only minor actors compared to government, employers, and the new entrepreneurial health care companies in leveraging and transforming the extant health care system. But restricted financial resources cannot explain their limited efforts to criticize the system or to point directions for future policy.

Foundations Today and Tomorrow

Foundations have considerable freedom to direct their activities at the same time that they are constrained by the mandate imposed by their founders, their prior experience, and the dominant forces in their environment. For example, the Duke Endowment, one of the major foundations with a commitment to health care activities, is restricted to making grants to institutions in North and South Carolina. In contrast, the Robert Wood Johnson Foundation, the largest supporter of health care activities among the foundations, decided early on to fund selected national programs, such as regional neonatal centers, inner-city community health centers, and school dental services, by soliciting competitive proposals and making awards to anywhere between five and fifty grantees, depending upon the specific program. Having found this mode of operation congenial, the foundation has gone far to institutionalize it.

As is true for every segment of the establishment (and foundations surely are part of the establishment), trustees and staff are careful to avoid activities that can lead to legal penalties or adverse publicity. Foundations must tread a narrow path between innovation and advocacy. Under the tax code, they risk their charitable status if they engage in political lobbying. Foundation staffs appreciate that the trustees who employ them expect to be protected from criticism and attack by others—politicians, professors, or the press. Hence, with the exception of the active opposition of a pro-life group to a foundation-supported health clinic offering family planning services at a school in the Midwest, it is difficult to identify any recent public attack on a major health foundation.

A review of the 1986 annual reports of the large foundations with strong health programs as well as a number of smaller organizations that focus almost all of their grant support on the health arena reveals a variety of programmatic emphases.

Education. Most of the larger foundations, as well as some of the smaller ones, direct a sizable proportion of their health care awards to talented young individuals to permit them to enhance their educational qualifications and to provide support for their research careers. Several foundations are particularly sensitive to the need to assist members of minority groups who are underrepresented in medicine to become practicing physicians, faculty members, and researchers. Closely related but still distinguishable are the interests of several foundations in the arena of health policy research. They offer funding to educate and train physicians and other medical personnel as health analysts possessing a broadened understanding of how political, social, and economic factors interact with and help to shape the changing contours of our health care system.

One step removed from the support of individuals, but still within the orbit of education, is foundation support of curriculum revision and reform or, more broadly, for restructuring health professional education in light of changing societal needs. These efforts cover a wide range, from the Henry J. Kaiser Family Foundation's support for the New Pathway Program at Harvard Medical School to the Pew Charitable Trust's National Dental Education Program, which involves funding for twenty-one dental schools to "encourage strategic planning and institutional change and renewal among the nation's dental schools." The Josiah Macy, Jr. Foundation, a relatively small philanthropy with a long-term focus on the medical arena, has in recent decades concentrated on "supporting and improving medical education" (at a level of $3.7 million in 1985–86). Much of its effort is directed to increasing the flow of minority students into careers in medicine, biomedical science, and related health professions.

Another activity related to education is a five-year project (1982–1987) of the Commonwealth Fund. The project assisted the nation's academic health centers to carry out their long-term missions of graduate medical education, specialized patient care, clinical research, and the care of uninsured patients in the face of intensified competition and the elimination of cross-subsidization by hospitals.

Populations at risk. Many foundations in the health field, with the Robert Wood Johnson Foundation in the lead, have directed sizable resources over several decades to improving the delivery of health care to various populations at risk, in particular low income-groups, people who live in underserved areas, newborns requiring costly and prolonged care, trauma victims, the homeless, patients discharged from mental hospitals, and others. The aim and expectation underlying such foundation support has been the development of successful models that could be widely replicated. Sometimes these expectations of replication have been realized, oftentimes not.

The rising national consciousness of the increasing numbers of elderly persons, many of them suffering from chronic illness and the frailties of age, has stimulated increasing foundation support. The John A. Hartford Foundation in its Aging and Health Program has identified the following priority areas for grant-making: improving the organization and financing of long-term care, medications problems of the elderly, and strengthening physicians' knowledge of geriatrics.

Health promotion and environmental health. The Henry J. Kaiser Family Foundation, after a two-year reevaluation of its grant-making strategy, decided to support a new major commitment to "health promotion" as well as a new emphasis on improving the results of health care "in ways that enhance the patients' functioning in their everyday lives." One of the oldest but also one of the smallest of the health foundations—the Milbank Memorial Fund, with a long-term commitment to public health—is phasing out its five-year program of clinical epidemiology fellowships for talented young physicians and has selected environmental occupational health as the focus of its future grant-making, starting with a hard look at the health problems of migratory farm workers.

Other activities. Three of the nation's largest foundations—the Ford Foundation, the W. K. Kellogg Foundation, and the John D. and Catherine T. MacArthur Foundation—pursue quite distinctive approaches in the health arena. In the case of Ford, health is not an explicit program area, although the foundation has made and continues to make significant amounts of money available for health-related activities via programs addressing population problems, including reproductive biology, and also in connection with its grants for the elimination of rural poverty in developing countries. The Kellogg Foundation, whose distinctive mission is "the application of knowledge to the problems of people," has focused much of its efforts on the area of health, which it sees as the "prerequisite to human well-being." Of its total grant program amounting to more than $80 million in 1986, the largest proportion was awarded to health (36 percent of total program grants), primarily for health promotion initiatives and the prevention of illness. The MacArthur Foundation disbursed more than $63 million in 1985; over $11 million went to health grants, heavily concentrated in the areas of mental health and the biology of parasitic diseases.

In 1985 the Andrew W. Mellon Foundation appropriated just under $65 million. Of this sum, higher education was the leading beneficiary, receiving $27 million. Medicine, public health, and population came next with grants of $17 million. Three-year awards totaling $5.35 million were made to fifteen major private medical schools, to finance junior faculty appointments for a number of able young scientists and to carry them to a point where they can compete independently for research support.

It should be noted that the Carnegie and Rockefeller foundations, which took the lead early in the century to move American medicine in new directions, had become minor actors in 1986. Among the later players were two with an almost exclusive focus on the support of biomedical research: the Howard Hughes Medical Institute, with prospective annual allocations of $300 million for the foreseeable future, and the Lucille P. Markey Charitable Trust, which made awards in excess of $45 million in 1986. The Markey Trust must dispose of its entire corpus, amounting to about $300 million (and more if the price of oil rises) by 1997.

In sum, present foundation giving for health is directed toward demonstrations aimed at improving the delivery of services to various (largely underserved) groups; assisting young health professionals to enhance their competences across a broad arena, from health policy to biomedical research; exploring alternative treatment and care modalities for the elderly; the reorientation of medicine to disease prevention and health promotion; and various approaches aimed at restructuring the delivery system to constrain costs.

Recommendations for Future Support

Since foundation funds amount to only 0.2 percent of all funds flowing into the health care system, I believe that foundations should exercise caution in their enthusiasm for small- or large-scale demonstrations directed at improving the delivery of health care. Such demonstrations are costly; many do not prove themselves, and replication is difficult. I would favor the reallocation of some part of these funds to the planning and policy arenas, with particular emphasis on assessing the strengths and weaknesses of different dimensions of the existing system and determining how weak links could be strengthened and new links put in place. We need more knowledge about the key facets of the existing system, and we need to use such knowledge to inform policy at every level—governmental, institutional, and individual.

Continuing operational issues. I have noted a number of "operational" issues that have been on the nation's agenda for a long time, although progress in grappling with them has been notoriously slow. One of these is the failure of many low-income women to seek early prenatal care, even when access is available. This confounds deeply held assumptions concerning the use of medical care and of preventive care services in particular. A clear understanding the specific barriers confronting this population is necessary to make for progress in improving the health of these women and the life chances of their infants.

A number of groups have been identified as failing to receive adequate essential health care services: inner-city low-income populations; rural low-income white and black populations; nursing home patients; and the seriously disabled and frail elderly who are homebound. Yet there is little specific information to indicate what are the most serious deficiencies in the experiences of each in obtaining access to care.

Though the explicit rationing of care has never been sanctioned by our society and its health care system, much has been said about the operation of implicit rationing. What can be learned from Medicare and other databases concerning the rationing of care by type of patient, location of hospital, and quality of staff?

Iatrogenic (treatment-induced) illness and premature death from improper use of prescription drugs and substandard performance in medical practice have achieved prominence in the context of malpractice litigation, soaring malpractice insurance rates, and their effects on style of practice and the crisis of care. But the underlying issue of the reasons for such evidences of malfunctions in medical practice and what can be done to reduce their frequency have, paradoxically, not been well studied. A related problem is the known existence of a substantial number of impaired physicians who remain in active practice and the ineffectiveness of existing mechanisms of control and discipline. Can alternative approaches be identified that are worth pursuing?

The "second opinion" mechanism has been in operation for about a decade in an effort to contain costs and to discourage risks that are engendered by unnecessary surgery. Is it not time to undertake a systematic assessment of the outcomes and the efficacy of this approach that is being increasingly used by payers for care?

Strategic policy issues. Equally important is the need for foundation support to improve the nation's capacity to understand and act on problems that have recently been put on its health agenda or soon will be. Now that the AMA has acknowledged the existence of a physician surplus, it surely is time that we explore alternative approaches to a problem that will require the involvement of state legislators, the medical establishment, and other parties. To continue to ignore the issues will only compound the difficulties of finding sensible solutions.

It is widely believed that our hospital plant has at least 200,000 excess beds. There has been no close look at this problem since it first surfaced about a decade ago. The public and others who pay hospital bills—government and private employers—need an up-to-date assessment of the facts. How much does an empty bed raise per diem costs? What are the preferred ways to respond if it is found that a large number of beds should be decertified and many hospitals merged or closed? With the cost of hospital care running in excess of $200 billion annually, it is unreasonable to continue to ignore the question of overcapacity.

With 40 million uninsured patients and with tens of millions of others having inadequate coverage, there are signs that the present system of private/public financing may soon enter the danger zone where it must be radically restructured. The opinion polls tell us that many Americans look favorably on the prospect of national health insurance, even though they have no comprehension of what such a system might imply for their continued access to quality health care. That is all the more reason, while there is still time, to explore alternative financing systems and to initiate a public dialogue.

Although many foundations have become interested in the

health problems of the elderly, many tough issues have not yet attracted the attention they deserve. These include the question of how to reduce the need for institutionalization, how to use both private and public funds to pay for long-term care without bankrupting families, and how to draw the distinction between socioeconomic and health needs in planning for older persons.

There is growing unease among both informed physicians and intelligent laypersons that the indiscriminate application of high technology at birth and at the end of life may be in conflict with, if it does not violate, the Hippocratic injunction to "do no harm." We need follow-up studies of the quality of life of congenitally disabled infants who are now being saved, just as we need careful studies of severely ill patients who are kept on life sustaining supports. These are admittedly difficult inquiries to pursue and even more difficult issues on which to reach a societal consensus. But in the absence of more reliable information and education, the public will continue to flounder.

The operational and strategic policy issues identified above are no more than a preliminary identification of areas that are worthy of foundation consideration and support. With additional time and reflection, some would probably be eliminated and others certainly added.

Dilemmas and Escape

Early in this century, foundation efforts in the health arena were future-oriented: transforming medical education; expanding basic and clinical research to improve the education and practice of physicians; ridding the nation of public health hazards. Most foundations today are oriented more to the present than to the future. Part of the explanation lies in the relatively modest means at their disposal to reshape the present very large, very complex, and very costly system. But I believe that there are additional forces that affect foundation policy. Foundations are loath to tangle with government; nevertheless, government funds over two-fifths of the system. Government needs strong and continuing critique by informed outsiders who are not seeking to gain specific advantages for any specific interest group. Further, private-sector funders and providers—accounting for another 30 percent of all expenditures—also need to be subjected to incisive critiques. Most foundation trustees and staff, however, do not see their mission as making big waves. The most serious inhibitor of basic reform is the academic establishment, which to a large extent provides the officers and the foot soldiers for the proposals that foundations fund. Academicians are as much a part of the establishment as foundation trustees and staff—possibly more so.

Probably the best escape from the dilemma of excessive caution that I have just outlined would be for the foundations, individually and possibly collectively, to establish over time a limited number of policy centers with directors of outstanding ability and to make a commitment to each of operating funds for ten years, subject to a five-year review. Such financial security would encourage these centers to address important, not mundane, problems. Even if only some of the directors rose to the challenge, I believe that the nation's health agenda would be advanced and that foundations would get a better run for their money than if they continue to parcel it out to a much larger number of worthy causes.

8

The Community Health Care Center

In 1977 the Robert Wood Johnson Foundation took the bold step of launching a large-scale demonstration of public, community-based health care delivery to inner-city residents. This effort was a logical extension of its commitment to expand access for the underserved groups in our society. The foundation identified the growing indigent population of the nation's urban centers as a persistent challenge to the health care system, despite more than a decade of liberally funded entitlement and service-delivery efforts by the federal government with the assistance of the states. It further recognized the critical role of local government, not only in the implementation of solutions — if solutions were to be found—but more fundamentally in the definition of problems and priorities, the design and redesign of systems, and the planning of actions that could translate programs into service delivery. This was the genesis of the Municipal Health Services Program (MHSP), a five-year effort to which the Johnson Foundation committed $15 million, that provided incentives for municipal governments to take the initiative in improving health care for their underserved residents.[1]

Specifically, the foundation offered substantial grants to five of the fifty largest cities in the United States for the implementation of proposals that seemed likely to improve the delivery of primary care to the poor, and to be sustainable by the locality at the termination of a five-year period of support. This goal was to be achieved though structural reform of the existing system, rather than the further proliferation of provider institutions and agencies. In fact, the segmentation of health care delivery for the poor was viewed as a systemic obstacle to meeting adequately their general medical care needs.

To provide maximum scope for the development of proposals that would have a substantial impact within each of the participating cities, the foundation did not commit the program to any specific model and stipulated only a few basic goals and assumptions. These included the development of community-based centers, located in identifiably underserved neighborhoods, that would offer a comprehensive array of services—including both the categorical services of public health departments and the general medical care available through the municipal hospitals' outpatient departments. This blending of resources was to be achieved in each city by the consolidation and elaboration of existing services, and was to be planned and carried out as a cooperative undertaking between the department of public health and the hospital department, under the direct leadership of the mayor. Moreover, it was anticipated that the program would entail no incremental costs to the locality, or at least none that could not be sustained at the end of the five-year demonstration period. Foundation support, amounting to $3 million per city, was intended to meet planning and start-up costs of the demonstration.

The many difficulties that confronted such an undertaking were evident from the outset: the receding ability (and interest) of local governments to address the service problems of the poor after a decade or more of aggressive federal leadership; the political powerlessness of the clientele that would use community health clinics, and a corresponding lack of responsiveness on the part of local political leadership; the potential political problems that might be invoked through competition with the few private practitioners serving low-income neighborhoods; the bureaucratic isolation and antagonisms of health departments and local municipal hospitals that would militate against the shift of patients from emergency rooms and outpatient departments of public hospitals to neighborhood clinics; and the difficulties of stretching and supplementing current revenues to effect a substantial increase in the quantity and quality of services for a substantial number of citizens, most of whom could not pay out-of-pocket for their care.[2]

Despite such substantial risk factors, the Johnson Foundation was encouraged to undertake the program by the willingness of the U.S. Conference of Mayors and the American Medical Association to cosponsor the effort. In addition to confirming explicitly the importance of the project, this collaboration offered support on two critical fronts: endorsement by the Conference of Mayors assured the active interest of the chief elected official in each of the cities, and thus materially enhanced the chances of success; and involvement of the AMA could help garner support from local physicians and moderate their concerns over the issue of competition.

A third collaborator, subsequently recruited, was the Health Care Financing Administration of the Department of Health and Human Services. By authorizing waivers for both Medicare and Medicaid programs—thus expanding the scope of benefits the centers could provide (particularly to the elderly) free of copayment—HCFA extended important financial resources to the MHSP demonstration sites and encouraged their utilization. HCFA further contributed by providing a sizable grant to Ronald Andersen, director of the Center for Health Administration Studies at the University of Chicago, to evaluate the changes in utilization and costs resulting from the MHSP demonstrations, and thereby establish the knowledge base for assessing their potential for replication. The findings of this study have been published.[3]

In parallel, the Robert Wood Johnson Foundation provided for a concurrent evaluation of the program by Conservation of Human Resources (CHR) at Columbia University. The CHR effort was designed to monitor the implementation process in each city and to assess the elements that facilitated or impeded the structural changes specified in the proposal. The legislative, bureaucratic, professional, and community dimensions of the project were the foci for this evaluation effort.

This chapter sets forth in summary form the CHR assessment of the MHSP effort. It then addresses the intrinsic policy issue— the potential of community health centers to provide affordable primary care for low-income, inner-city populations.

Assessment of the Demonstration Project

Overview. Of the nation's 50 largest cities eligible to participate in the demonstration project, 28 submitted formal proposals, and 5 were awarded grants: Baltimore, Cincinnati, Milwaukee, St. Louis, and San Jose. The variability among these sites is immediately apparent: the cities differ in their geography, economy, population, sociopolitical characteristics, governance, and history, to say nothing of the structure and functioning of their health care systems. Their proposals clearly reflected these differences and, while pursuing a common goal, ranged widely in substance. Cincinnati's project aimed to expand the service program of a preexistent citywide network of traditional categorical clinics and improve their operations through the introduction of a computerized information system. Milwaukee proposed to locate and coordinate its entire gamut of social welfare services at several multiservice sites. St. Louis wished to transform a historic set of preventive care-oriented health department clinics, managed and staffed by public health nurses, to fit a primary care medical model. Baltimore proposed to eliminate gradually its publicly operated services in favor of a variety of subsidized group-practice arrangements. In San Jose the funds were to be used to expand the health service programs and capacities of a number of independent community-based organizations.

The development and structure of health care services for the urban poor in each of these cities is described in a baseline study prepared as the first part of the CHR evaluation. The report, *Health Care for the Urban Poor*, which appeared in 1983, reviews critically the major federal health policy initiatives from the Johnson administration on, focusing on their impact upon ambulatory care for the indigent, and examines the history and literature of community health care centers (CHCs).[4] A systematic reconstruction of the successive stages of the demonstration and a wealth of operating data and detailed process information describing its progress are presented and analyzed thematically in a second volume, published in 1985, entitled *Local Health Policy in Action: The Municipal Health Services Program*.[5] Accordingly, this chapter will summarize briefly the success and shortcomings of the program in terms of the explicit goals of its sponsors; it will then turn to a discussion of the program's implications for the future role of CHCs, and consider alternative policies for providing health care to the indigent.

Achievements of the demonstration. The establishment and elaboration of neighborhood health centers for the provision of ambulatory care to the inner-city poor which would prove to be a feasible and desirable alternative to the municipal hospital was the principal goal of the demonstration, and the record unequivocally confirms its achievement. Each city succeeded in implementing the proposed number and variety of clinic programs and, in fact, each added sites beyond the three required by the foundation. At its peak, four years into the program, 21 clinics were in operation, although subsequent closings and a substitution reduced the final count to 19; two cities operated three sites, two operated four, and one (Baltimore) operated five.

The associated objective, to enhance the quality of ambulatory care through an integrated program of preventive and therapeutic services, was also accomplished. Clinics that had previously been restricted to traditional public health functions or the provision of categorical services such as maternal and child care were transformed into comprehensive health centers that were available to the entire local population. In at least two of the cities, MHSP effected a basic reorientation of the service delivery goals and methods of a well-entrenched clinic system, run along classic lines by the department of health, that long antedated the comprehensive community efforts of the 1960s. In two others, the program components included the expansion and redirection of existing ambulatory care providers concurrently with the establishment of new primary care centers with a broader health mission. The conversion from one model to another engendered varying degrees of conflict among bureaucracies and professional sectors, but these older clinics retained the support of their patient clientele and built up to target utilization goals more readily than the newly established facilities, which had to develop their enrollment slowly. The overall receptivity of patients to neighborhood-based care is reflected in the clinics' utilization statistics; in the course of five years the annual number of visits more than quadrupled, from 100,000 to over 450,000.[6]

A second major goal of the program, to effect a fundamental organizational reform in the health care delivery system by reducing and perhaps ultimately eliminating the role of the hospital as a source of primary care, turned out to be more problematic. While the neighborhood centers succeeded in enrolling patients who had formerly been treated in outpatient clinics and emergency rooms of both municipal and voluntary hospitals, there was no evidence of a substantial decline in the utilization of these facilities as a result of the MHSP demonstration. Accordingly, there was no significant redeployment of either financial or staff resources from hospitals to community clinics. As for systemic quality improvement through new arrangements between the community clinics and the hospitals for the provision of subspecialty and inpatient care, the anticipated staff linkages did not materialize and the familiar duplications and discontinuities resulting from this dualism persisted, at least in the case of patients needing services that were beyond the scope of the community center.

Achievement of the third major objective—viability of the centers after termination of the subsidy—was equivocal. The analysis of the cost data leaves no doubt that the cost per visit at the community center was much below that at ambulatory units of public hospitals, whether an emergency room or a general outpatient clinic. In the final year, cost per visit ranged from $31 to $65, with an average of $57 (exclusive of the central administrative unit). In no city did the clinic cost exceed 50 percent of the public hospital outpatient cost; the range was from 24 to 50 percent, and the average, 39 percent. This difference could have been related to differences in case and service mix between the MHSP clinics and the hospital outpatient departments. Even at peak operations, all the clinics remained dependent (to a greater or lesser degree) on the Johnson Foundation grant money and on revenues from the Medicare waiver. In the final year of the program, operating deficits averaged 13 percent of clinic expenses, and foundation support covered from 9 to 22 percent of the individual clinic's budget. Medicare contributed an average of 30 percent of total clinic costs. In three of the cities, those with the highest costs, Medicare contributed from 30 to 81 percent of revenues, and from 26 to 72 percent of expenses. The remaining two cities depended upon Medicare for 6 to 15 percent of their costs and 7 to 19 percent of their revenues, respectively. Reductions in the scope of services and restoration of conventional Medicare copayment requirements will inevitably cause a diminution in the number of revenue-producing patient visits, which will be critical in all but one or at the most two of the cities. In addition, the expectation that the clinics would enroll a fair number of privately insured patients and others able to pay some part of their costs was not realized.

The need for further subsidy via local tax funds suggests that the survival of the individual clinics will be contingent upon their political support. Most will continue to operate in some form, very likely at a reduced level. Hence the viability of the MHSP centers at the end of the demonstration was uncertain.

Key ancillary findings from MHSP. A number of findings either confirmed or challenged the assumptions that undergirded the demonstration and that have long guided the search for health system reforms to benefit the poor.

(1) The sites chosen by the municipality for participation in the program were located in neighborhoods that had been identified as seriously bereft of health resources and manifesting high indices of ill health, implying a lack of access to needed health care services. However, a concurrent survey found the number and proportion of the targeted inner-city population with no regular source of care to be considerably smaller than had originally been believed. Many of the poor and near poor continued to obtain some or all of their care from private practitioners located in and especially adjacent to low-income areas.

(2) While the MHSP did reach those who had previously been served by the emergency room and outpatient clinics of the public hospital, many continued to seek care from these facilities, notwithstanding distance and inconvenience, even after services became available at the neighborhood health center.

(3) Both the new and expanded community health centers were able over the years to increase their utilization to a level at which the calculated unit costs of the services they provided were considerably below the costs of an ambulatory care visit at the municipal hospital.

(4) The ability of the centers to provide both preventive and therapeutic services within the same setting was a boon to patients, particularly to mothers with young children and to the elderly, although in all but one city the MHSP patient population did not contain large proportions of the elderly or chronically ill.

(5) The financial viability of the centers depended in large measure on the foundation's subvention and on the additional revenues generated by the Medicare and Medicaid waivers. The centers had little success in attracting private patients with insurance or the ability to pay out-of-pocket.

(6) It was not feasible to shift the patient load and treatment resources from the municipal hospital to the community health centers, as the project design had contemplated. Although those individuals who used the MHSP received less outpatient and emergency room care, the total volume of ambulatory services to the city's poor increased. There is some evidence of a reduction in the utilization of inpatient care by MHSP patients, although its magnitude and certainty are statistically limited.

(7) Since most of the funding for the centers derived from state, federal, and foundation sources, the mayor proved to be a less powerful force for reform than had initially been assumed. In three of the five cities, control and operation of the public hospital were outside the jurisdiction of the municipality, and this seriously constrained the mayor's leverage to restructure services and to reallocate resources.

The Changing Environment of Community Health Centers

The implicit purpose of any social experiment is to provide generalizable lessons that can be translated into broader policy formulation. Can we extrapolate from the experience of the five demonstration projects to formulate directions for a public policy that will assure that health services to the urban poor are maintained and indeed improved in the changing health care environment? And if this is the way to go, what concomitant adjustments should be made in the extant delivery system, and how can they be accomplished?

It must be stated at the outset that the assessment of the MHSP does not yield unequivocal findings that point in a single policy direction. The variability among the five demonstration sites with respect to such key factors as size of the population in need, preexisting health resources, political leadership, and financial capability clearly argues against definitive findings and uniform recommendations.

A second reason for the inability of the assessment to yield conclusive policy directions, is endemic to all social experiments: the difficulty of evaluating the effects of intervening in a nonconstant experimental field. During the life of the demonstration and the years immediately following, the health care environment underwent radical transformation. Of the major

developments that have occurred, some might have been anticipated, but others clearly could not. For example, the demand
for health care services moderated at a time when increasing
numbers of physicians were entering practice and the nation's
hospitals had to contend with a large number of vacant beds.[7]
Second, advances in medical knowledge and technology, reinforced by cost pressures, have resulted in the shift of a large
volume of treatment to ambulatory settings and a further reduction in the demand for patient care.[8] On another front, a change
in the political climate at both federal and state levels has led
to tax ceilings and tax reductions and thus diminished the funding available for social welfare programs, including appropriations for Medicaid.[9] Finally, new forms of health care delivery,
in particular, prepayment plans, propose to provide acceptable
care at an affordable price.[10]

These forces have variously and interactively affected the
course, the form, and the outcome of the MHSP, by revealing
the presence of a larger number of providers interested in caring
for the poor than had originally been assumed, by suggesting
alternatives to the public ambulatory care facility, by evoking
contending health issues of wide public concern—such as the
endangered inner-city hospital—and by severely weakening
some of the sources of financial support on which the program
relied.

Just as these changes influenced the outcome of the MHSP,
future changes will affect the outcome of alternative policies
designed to meet the objective of acceptable, affordable care for
the urban poor. Undoubtedly, the health care system to which
these policies will be addressed will be significantly altered over
the next decade, although estimates differ about the specificity,
the magnitude, and the rate of these alterations. Following are
some of the more probable changes:

Many of the nation's largest cities will continue to experience
a decline in the size of their populations. The number of inner-
city poor may stabilize or even decrease in cities with 500,000
to 1,500,000 inhabitants. Nevertheless, it is a virtual demographic certainty that considerable numbers of inner-city residents will continue to need access to no-cost and low-cost health
services.

The nation's supply of physicians, which amounted to 140 per

100,000 population in 1950 and is now nearing the 220 mark, will probably reach 260 per 100,000 by 1995, and may go even higher than that.[11]

The federal government, which currently contributes more than half of the funds for Medicaid, faces a steadily increasing budgetary stringency, and this almost certainly assures efforts to constrain future outlays for health entitlement programs, both Medicaid and Medicare. The states too will aim to control their expenditures for health care, since Medicaid has represented one of the fastest-growing components of their budgets. Paradoxically, several states have recently expanded access to their Medicaid programs in the wake of popular demand for coverage of the indigent.[12]

The introduction of DRGs, the growth of for-profit medical enterprises, and the concerns of employers to limit the costs of employee health care coverage are among the many new forces that are making the health care market more competitive and more price-sensitive. Inner-city voluntary hospitals which historically provided a considerable volume of charity care, particularly ambulatory services, are under increasing pressure to cut back as they face a more competitive environment.[13]

In response to mounting pressures from the purchasers of insurance to restrain their premium outlays, commercial insurance companies are moving aggressively to reduce the practice of cross-subsidization, which has in the past enabled many voluntary hospitals to cover some of the cost of unreimbursed services to the poor.[14]

The dampening demand for health care and the increasing numbers of physicians and excess beds have stimulated many providers to explore new delivery systems that aim to "lock in" a steady flow of insured patients. Even Medicaid patients present a potentially attractive market to many providers.[15]

All of these trends are likely to be strengthened in the decade ahead. There are, in addition, other factors with less certain but significant impact on the health care environment.

A large stream of immigrants, legal and illegal, enter the United States each year; most of them locate in urban centers, and most of them are poor and will remain poor during their initial years here. What is more, many present or contract health problems that, if neglected, are a danger to them and to others in their environment. Illegal immigrants threatened with apprehension and deportation generally avoid (except in emergency) seeking care in public facilities.[16] It is uncertain to what extent the revised immigration statutes of 1986 will succeed in moderating the large-scale inflow.

The rate of economic growth, the major determinant of the demand for labor, will have a significant impact on the rate of immigration, on individual and family incomes, and on the tax revenues of the various levels of government. Although optimists are sanguine about our expanding economy, others believe it is imperiled by foreign and internal debts. If an economic slow-down should develop and persist for a number of years, the problems of meeting the health care needs of the urban poor will be compounded.

While the Health Insurance Trust Fund will not face bankruptcy for at least ten to fifteen years and is therefore less of a pressing issue than it recently has been, there is broad agreement in both Congress and the White House that Medicare costs should be reduced. The administration favors larger user payments and increased deductibles, while the Congress favors a reimbursement freeze or cutback. It seems likely that the elderly will pay more and hospitals and physicians will receive less in the future.[17]

Demonstrations are under way in various parts of the country aimed at enrolling both Medicaid and Medicare beneficiaries in prepayment plans, which purport to control costs and at the same time provide patients with more appropriate care. It is too early to assess the potential of these approaches. However, no prepayment plan is likely to succeed unless it can be protected from the financial consequences of adverse selection. In the case of voluntary enrollment of Medicare beneficiaries, capitation rates will have to be adjusted to reflect the actuarial experience of the elderly.[18] With respect to Medicaid eligibles, the failure of the Commonwealth Health Care Corporation, Boston's well-designed prepaid health care program for Medicaid beneficiaries, has demonstrated the value that many low-income persons place on retaining freedom of choice of providers.[19] Nevertheless, several states have moved to limit provider options for Medicaid enrollees, and others are likely to follow.

A number of states—among them New York, New Jersey,

Massachusetts, and Florida—have established a hospital support system designed to create a pool of revenue dollars which is redistributed among the member providers in proportion to their charity cases and bad debts. This approach offers the prospect of enabling voluntary hospitals with a long commitment to the urban poor to continue to serve them without risking insolvency.[20]

The future role of local governments in providing for the health care needs of the poor is a formidable unknown. They appear to be withdrawing gradually from active hospital operation, the historic function of local government, by a number of routes: straightforward termination and closure; sale to a for-profit chain (with some guarantees for admission of the indigent); and occasionally transfer of the municipal hospital to a nonprofit sponsor (as in Baltimore).[21] Such actions have been more frequent in smaller communities, but there have been instances where city or county government in a large metropolitan area has ceased to provide hospital care. As between political pressures to keep public hospitals operating and budgetary pressures to relieve local government of the burden of escalating hospital expenditures, the future balance is uncertain.

The Future of the Urban Community Health Center

Having delineated both the probable trends and the uncertainties in the health care environment, we can now address the central policy question: what would be the preferred way for urban communities to provide an acceptable level of ambulatory care to their inner-city poor in the decade ahead? More specifically, what should be the role of community health care centers in the evolving urban health care system?

Although it was a major programmatic initiative of the Great Society, the effort to establish a nationwide network of community health care centers never realized its ambitious goal of becoming the preferred provider of ambulatory care to inner-city populations. What is more, even after Medicare and Medicaid reimbursement became available, few of these centers were able to achieve and maintain financial independence. Almost all have had to rely, to a greater or lesser degree, on annual subsidies. In terms of their operations, it is evident that many community health care centers now provide a desirable level of care in convenient locations to inner-city families, and that these centers have been able to attract and retain a satisfied patient clientele—a fact that is supported by the experience of the five-city MHSP demonstration. The first question, then, is whether, in a period of persisting financial stringency, existing centers should continue to be subsidized.

Part of the answer must be pragmatic. If a community has high regard for its health care centers, if large numbers of the neighborhood residents are satisfied with the services they receive, and if the government and/or philanthropy can be persuaded to meet their annual deficits, there is good reason for the centers to continue operating.

A more complicated policy choice arises if the level of funding for both the municipal hospital and the community health centers is cut back, and total inpatient and ambulatory care capacity must be reduced. Current trends in medical care and in public administration suggest that a reduction in the number of inpatient beds would be the preferred first-order accommodation. The second-order response would be to identify those ambulatory care facilities that could most readily be contracted or eliminated, based on location and user preferences. The experience of the MHSP has indicated that, other things being equal, the cost of ambulatory care in the neighborhood centers is considerably less than that of emergency room and outpatient care at the public hospital. But other things are often not equal: neighborhood centers are unable to provide emergency care for trauma and to treat ambulatory patients with complicated diseases. As long as it remains necessary to operate the municipal hospital as a provider of last resort, the preferred choice may be to close one or more neighborhood centers, particularly if their level of utilization is low.

The conclusion that logic justifies the continued support of effectively functioning community health care centers does not, however, imply support for their further proliferation. We have noted that the population in many inner cities is more likely to remain stable or even decline than to increase. In light of the finding of the MHSP survey that as long as five years ago few inner-city residents lacked access to health care, it is reasonable to conclude that future demand will increase little, if at all, and could decline. In such an environment there is no compelling need for the establishment of new centers. It may be advantageous, however, to provide service programs of broader scope and better quality in the existing community health centers, under conditions conducive to greater utilization. MHSP patient loads expanded rapidly in response to the introduction of new services, preventive and therapeutic, as the result of the foundation grant and the Medicare and Medicaid waivers.

Extension of the waiver by the federal government for the centers that participated in the MHSP has been conditioned upon the development and adoption of a capitation system. Since few cities have moved in this direction, the centers are more likely to face a cutback than an expansion in the range of the services they will be able to offer. It is possible that centers that have enrolled a substantial number of Medicare beneficiaries and other patients with incomes above poverty level will be able to continue to offer some of the waivered services on a fee-for-service basis or through a prepayment arrangement.

Alternatives to the community health care centers. Several alternative sources hold substantial promise of supplementing the community health care centers over the next ten years. First, in a decade which will see a rapidly increasing supply of physicians, it is likely that some new entrants into the profession will explore the feasibility of establishing a group practice in or near an inner-city neighborhood.[22] Since such independent practice arrangements can provide ambulatory care services to patients at an average visit cost considerably below that of most community health centers, they should be favored over a plan for center expansion. This recommendation, however, does not preclude support for the establishment of new center in a neighborhood with no ready access to ambulatory care and where physicians, either individually or as members of a group, are unwilling to locate. In the absence of practitioners and with no hospital in the vicinity, a new center—particularly one that has substantial community approval—may well offer the best opportunity to improve access to needed health care services.

Inner-city voluntary hospitals themselves recognize that they face a dwindling inpatient census and need to ensure for themselves a constant referral pool. Some institutions are devising programs for the delivery of ambulatory care services at satellite locations, including neighborhood health centers, with the expectation that these will enable the hospital to optimize its inpatient load.[23]

Such new departures in the provision of ambulatory care, currently in demonstration form if not in full-blown operation, could evolve into viable delivery modes for the inner city. Each year is likely to see further innovations, now that patients with public entitlements are becoming more attractive to the swollen ranks of physicians and to hospitals experiencing census declines, and governments are attempting to slow or even cap the growth of their health care expenditures. In this environment, there is a continuing place for established community health centers that are operating close to the break-even point. There are even the preconditions to justify some additional centers in spite of the desire of government to avoid new outlays for health care. But unless the American economy experiences a vigorous growth for the next five to ten years that is reflected in strong demand for labor, sizable gains in personal income, and enlarged government revenues—an unlikely but not impossible scenario—it is reasonable to expect shrinkage in the number of existing centers, and a reduction in the range of services that they provide. Only an occasional new center is likely to be established.

The Uninsured Population

The preceding analyses and recommendations have focused primarily on inner-city health centers that treat Medicare and Medicaid patients, for whom they receive reimbursement. Operating data from the MHSP indicate, however, that many people who use these centers have no third-party coverage at all, and are able to pay only part of their charges at most. The MHSP centers failed to attract sufficient numbers of patients with private insurance to generate the excess revenue needed to help offset the costs of such unreimbursed care. The inability to cover with patient revenues alone the free or below-cost care that they provide for the uninsured is a primary reason why even established, efficiently operated community health centers have been dependent—some more, some less—on subsidies.

Since the passage of Medicaid in 1965, the care of the uninsured poor has been met differently in different cities—by municipal or county hospitals, by local voluntary hospitals that have a tradition of serving the poor, by community health centers (usually with the assistance of government and philanthropic subsidies), or by other free-standing or satellite clinics. As voluntary hospitals have come under increasing financial pressure, the proportion of free care that they have been able to provide has declined, and more of the responsibility for the indigent has shifted to the public hospitals and the subsidized community health centers.[24] In an effort to maintain the number of providers willing to treat the uninsured poor, several states have in recent years moved (some with the help of waivers from HCFA) to establish all-payer systems which provide at least partial fiscal relief to institutions that perform substantial uncompensated service.[25] Prior to the implementation of this cooperative financing mechanism, New York and several other states had allocated special funds for the same purpose through a program known as "ghetto medicine."[26]

Other attempts are under way to explore the potential of "insuring" the uninsured with the help of state and private funds, the latter characteristically contributed jointly by third-party payers following some distributive formula. As various analyses have made clear, however, there are formidable difficulties in developing designs that do not lead to dysfunctional outcomes.[27]

The final alternative is one that in recent years has virtually disappeared from the nation's health agenda but may yet return; that is, one or another form of national health insurance which would provide some level of coverage for the entire population.[28] Under a program of universal coverage that would preserve the principle of freedom of choice that currently prevails in most of the health care system, community health centers could be strengthened and their financial viability secured by their ability to be compensated for the treatment of all their patients, including those currently unable to pay. It is simplistic, however, to assume that this would be the necessary outcome of national health insurance. Such a radical political and economic transformation would generate a great many other changes in health care delivery that could either strengthen or weaken the role of community health care centers. Not the least important in terms of the proliferation of CHCs as a preferred modality of care would be the relative availability of capital funds in a system providing universal benefits, and the allocation of those funds among different types of facilities.

The Potential of CHCs

Stimulated initially by federal money in the mid-1960s, community health centers have been established in inner cities throughout the country, although never in the number originally projected, and many have contributed substantially to providing improved primary care for low-income populations. Even the most efficiently operated centers have, almost without exception, been dependent on annual subsidies, partly because of the considerable volume of free care that they provide to the uninsured; their support in a straitened fiscal environment as the preferred modality of care for the indigent is a current issue for local government. In the case of a center that provides a significant volume of ambulatory care to a satisfied user population, and that requires an annual subsidy that is not an excessive burden to government and/or philanthropy, the preferred policy should be to support its continuing operation. Whenever feasible, the center should explore new relationships with local physician groups, with other ambulatory care facilities, and with nearby hospitals, both public and voluntary, in order to improve referral and follow-up arrangements that would result in more and better care at lower total costs.

In light of the stable or declining populations projected for many inner-city areas, the increasing pressures for fiscal restraint, and the growing numbers of physicians, a policy of caution should be followed with respect to the establishment of new community health centers; this does not imply blanket opposition to any additions. With a large number of young physicians seeking opportunities for practice, with considerable momentum in the direction of prepaid delivery systems, and with other innovative approaches to health care delivery, there are reasonable prospects that these alternatives may be able to provide more and better services at lower cost per patient. And, in a period of cutting costs, the public hospital with its emergency room and specialty clinics must remain as provider of last resort for the urban poor. Effective as community health centers are, they cannot substitute for the broader services of the public hospital and its specialty clinics. In sum, the future role of the community health center must be assessed not simply by its performance as an independent health care modality, but by its contribution to the totality of the health care system available to the urban poor.

Finally, it is important that private third-party payers and the local philanthropic leadership explore and support all-payer systems, which offer the best opportunity at this time (and probably for the decade ahead) for all providers—public, nonprofit, and private—to cooperate in the care of the poor and particularly the uninsured. If the costs of uncompensated care are not shared, an excessive burden will fall on the public sector; in a period of cost constraint this would inevitably lead to serious deterioration in the quantity and quality of services available to the urban poor.

Community health centers have contributed to improved ambulatory care for the urban poor, and with strong leadership they have the potential to make further contributions. But in the rapidly changing urban and medical care environment, the community health center represents only one of a number of alternatives and cannot be viewed as the sole or even the principal instrument for improving health care in the inner city.

9

Health Care in New York City

There are two ways of reading the tumultuous events that occurred on the health care front in New York City between 1964 and 1984. The first emphasizes the explosive rise in annual outlays, approximately $10 billion in inflation-free dollars, or almost threefold on a per capita basis. A second way of assessing this tumultuous period is to realize that despite the much-enlarged inflow of dollars, the underlying structure of health care delivery in the city remained largely intact. To oversimplify: most physicians continued to treat patients on a fee-for-service basis in private offices, where they practiced individually or in association with one or more colleagues. The large voluntary hospitals continued to be dominant providers of inpatient care for the majority of citizens, with the municipal hospitals attending to large numbers of the poor.

In 1984, as in 1964, the city could count six medical schools located within its borders, although in the interim New York Medical College had relocated to suburban Westchester County and the Mt. Sinai School of Medicine of the City University of New York opened its doors to students in 1968. The city's academic health centers continued to be in the forefront of both medical research and undergraduate and graduate medical education.

The National Context

There is a strong probability that the next decade—which will take us to the end of the century—will witness the play upon the U.S. health care system of powerful forces stemming from changes in financing, market structures, human resources, and consumer behavior, and these will be reflected in the structure of health care in New York City. While we cannot identify all of the forces, much less calculate their outcome precisely, we should be able to delineate the interactions between these over-arching or "macro" trends and the evolving health care struc-ture in New York City.

The voluntary hospitals, and in particular the large teaching affiliates of the six academic health centers, are the driving force of the health care delivery system in New York City. Their relative importance has increased in recent decades as many smaller proprietary and voluntary hospitals have closed; as the municipal hospital system has shrunk and has come to depend for its professional staff on contractual relations with affiliates in the voluntary sector; and as the large voluntary institutions have become responsible for a growing proportion of hospital-based ambulatory care in the city. One revealing clue to the dominance of the major teaching hospitals is their consistently high rate of occupancy during recent years.

The critical question is how these dominant institutions are likely to fare in the years ahead in the face of the DRGs, all-payer systems, the pressure for more treatment in ambulatory settings, cost increases stemming from the large capital expen-ditures, changes in referral patterns, and still other forces that may appear on the horizon.

Since 1980 several of the major academic health centers have filed with their states applications for certificates of need to rehabilitate and modernize their aging facilities, with strong expectations that they will continue to operate in the future much as they have in the past. Without exception, their original proposals to Albany assumed the maintenance of their present capacity with its strong bias in favor of inpatient services. Op-erating at the 90 percent occupancy level, there was no reason to scale back the number of their beds. Occupancy as a criterion is conditioned, however, upon the maintenance of revenue flows adequate to cover expenditures incurred for the given level of operations (with some surplus for innovation and improvements) if the institution is to retain solvency. The hospitals' planners may have given insufficient consideration to the powerful influences upon payers at present to depart from cost reimbursement and to restrict, if not eliminate, the opportunity for hospitals to cross-subsidize their operations by charging certain patients more, thus compensating for those who pay less. The action of the Congress in 1983 to institute DRGs as the basis for payment for Medicare patients, and the distinct possibility that all payers may sooner or later adopt the same approach, present a major financial threat to the voluntary hospitals in New York City.

Cost Cutting

The first and overriding contributory factor is the excessive length of stay in New York City hospitals (the highest in the country), which is approximately 40 percent above that of comparable large urban hospitals in California. Since the regional and national reimbursement rates for DRGs will be determined in large measure by the length of stay, New York City hospitals face the serious challenge of moving closer to the national norm, preferably dropping below the norm.

The average length has in fact been steadily decreasing in New York City, particularly in the municipal system, so there is some question about the remaining potential in this direction. To the extent, however, that the hospitals will succeed in achieving future reductions—and the pressure to do so will be severe—their bed requirements will moderate, probably substantially.

A strong reinforcing factor will come from the pressures that are building up from many sources to shift a greater volume of care from inpatient to ambulatory settings. In fact, many specialists believe that there are clear gains to the patient from such a shift and they are taking the lead to expand the practice of ambulatory surgery as well as complex diagnostic and therapeutic services. Payers are introducing economic incentives to accomplish the same end by agreeing to cover all the costs for ambulatory procedures but only part of the costs when the same procedures are performed in an inpatient setting.

Other factors that are likely to moderate the use of inpatient facilities are the expansion of enrollments in various prepaid delivery systems, which are associated with much-reduced hospital admission rates; the probability that Medicare beneficiaries will have to pay more out of pocket for inpatient care, which would tend to reduce their level of demand; and the intensified competition between the increased supply of physicians and hospitals, which will depress inpatient admissions. Further, as more and more competent physicians locate their practice in the suburbs, the number of referrals to the large teaching hospitals in the city will continue to decline. Finally, the increase of $100 or more in per diem rates to cover the costs of new construction will add one more hurdle to maintaining high occupancy rates in the major teaching hospitals in a period of fiscal constraint.

The counterview that would be more upbeat about the future of the voluntary hospitals in New York City would stress that they are currently operating on an all-payer system, and very likely will continue to do so in the future; that the rich pool of specialist talent in New York City will continue to draw sufficient numbers of patients from beyond the city's limits to keep occupancy rates high; that the above-average number of elderly among the city's population with their differentially higher admission rates will also contribute to the maintenance of high occupancy; and that the training of large numbers of residents, which will surely continue, also contributes to the greater use of hospital facilities.

No matter how the occupancy issue resolves itself, it is difficult to foresee any circumstances in which the principal teaching affiliate of each of the academic health centers will not continue to be the institution of choice for many patients in and out of the city. More problematic is the future of selected independent voluntary hospitals that have large indigent patient rolls and are in need of capital renovation. We know from the recent past that not all such institutions have survived, and if the financial environment should tighten, as we must anticipate, several other large voluntary hospitals may be at risk.

The Municipal Institution

The major municipal hospitals—Bellevue, Harlem, North Central Bronx, Bronx Municipal Hospital Center, Kings County, and Elmhurst—are in some cases so intricately intertwined with the operation of the several academic centers—Downstate, New York University, Columbia-Presbyterian, Mt. Sinai, and Einstein—and are so critical to the delivery of health care to large concentrations of low-income groups that it is difficult to foresee an imminent or even eventual closure of any of them. Their political-economic importance for the city's minority constituencies exercises an all-but-irresistible push against their elimination. As one senior government official observed of the politically traumatic termination of Sydenham Hospital, a small, inefficient facility of admittedly low quality, "This is the last hospital closure that I ever intend to be involved in and I doubt whether the city will soon attempt any more."

Since the occupancy rates in municipal hospitals have been in the 80 percent range, the major opportunity for the system to tighten its operation is to cut back its authorized capacity and to orient its capital plans to a modernized but smaller plant with expanded ambulatory care facilities when funds become available. That is the guideline for Kings County Hospital, which is among the first scheduled for reconstruction.

The last two decades have witnessed several conflicting trends with respect to the provision of ambulatory care. On the one hand, the dearth and ultimate disappearance of private practitioners in neighborhoods abandoned by the middle class has resulted in the dependence of their present residents, the poor, on the local hospital for ambulatory care. A counterdevelopment was the establishment and expansion of community health centers, which sought to provide a substitute for the vanishing private practitioner and the hospital emergency room. A second substitute was the development of for-profit practice groups oriented to the Medicaid population. In terms of scale, hospital-based ambulatory care represented by far the largest of the three approaches.

Health Maintenance Organizations

Although New York City has one of the oldest and largest of all prepaid health care systems in the country—the Health Insurance Plan (HIP)—it has not demonstrated much capacity for growth in recent decades. As of 1983, the heart of its membership of 867,000 consisted of municipal employees and the members of selected trade unions. Until recently, the city has not been an encouraging environment for the establishment and growth of new delivery systems. Early in 1974 Connecticut General established an HMO in Brooklyn, which failed to attract the minimal necessary enrollment, lost a considerable sum, and was accordingly short-lived. Blue Cross/Blue Shield has also sought to stimulate HMO development, but thus far its efforts have met with only limited success. Its own effort, the BC/BS of Greater New York HMO, has a membership of 52,000.

What has been responsible for the desultory growth of HMOs and the resistance of the city to new delivery systems? The explanation may be found in the preference of middle- and upper-income people to select their own physicians; the preference of most physicians for fee-for-service or hospital-based practice; the disinclination of major hospitals to provide back-up arrangements; and the difficulties of preventing HMO staff from engaging in private practice on the side. Probably the most important determinant is the inability to identify a site within the city accessible to a critical mass of younger middle-class families who would be the natural constituency of an HMO. This population is now diffused throughout the suburban counties. It should be noted that the last year covered in this chapter, 1985, has seen an upsurge of activity by numerous groups, voluntary and for-profit, to establish a variety of HMOs in the metropolitan area.

If one shifts focus from the middle class to the poor, one finds that they too have been hard to organize around a prepaid practice plan. One interesting experiment has been under way at Metropolitan; Montefiore has explored the potential of a prepaid plan in the South Bronx; and Governor Mario Cuomo is committed to initiating demonstration projects among the Medicaid population. A first effort undertaken conjointly with the mayor in East Harlem met resistance from the local population and from state and local legislators over the issue of "lock-ins" and the abrogation of "freedom of choice" for the poor.

In its 1984 spring legislative session New York State took two actions with respect to ambulatory care: it raised the reimbursement rate to voluntary hospitals for an emergency room visit from $60 to $70 and it increased the schedule of physician's fees for an office visit for Medicaid patients by 30 percent. It is questionable, however, that these actions of the legislature and the governor's expressed interest in stimulating enrollment of Medicaid patients in prepaid plans will effect major alterations in the existing patterns of ambulatory care during the next decade. Most middle-class residents will continue to seek care from private practitioners; most poor persons will continue to rely on the ambulatory facilities of neighborhood hospitals and to a lesser degree on community health centers, fee-for-service practitioner groups, and a small number of slow-growing prepaid practice organizations.

Other developments, however, may alter the foregoing. The combination of Medicare fiscal reforms, which substantially increased copayments by users and which made a voucher system a more attractive incentive to prepaid plans to enroll the elderly, could result in the accelerated growth of prepayment groups. One must also allow for the possibility that some hospitals will expand the range of their market penetration by moving to develop new financing and delivery arrangements that will include the provision of ambulatory care services on a prepaid or fee-for-service basis, or a combination of both. Moreover, some primary care services could be delivered at off-hospital sites, that is, in satellite clinics or by arrangement with designated groups of physicians practicing in the community.

There is no question that for-profit corporations specializing in ambulatory care—walk-in clinics, emergency care centers, surgi-centers—have extended beyond their initial centers of growth in the South and the West to open facilities in the Midwest, and are exploring opportunities in the Northeast, which until now has been an unfriendly market. The question that we face is whether the combination of the particular health care market in New York City and the strong regulatory structure in Albany will inhibit serious efforts by corporate medicine to establish a presence in New York City. In this connection it is well to recall that for-profit nursing homes were able to grow rapidly in the New York City area at the same time that many proprietary hospitals were forced to close their doors.

Care for the Elderly

In addition to the growth of private nursing home beds, the last decades have seen the expansion of nonprofit nursing home capacity, as well as a substantial government effort to care for Medicaid patients in their own homes, and recent experimental programs (the "Nursing Home Without Walls" championed by State Senator Tarky Lombardi is an example) that provide community-based services aimed at reducing prospective admissions of middle-class and Medicaid patients to nursing homes.

Despite widespread belief to the contrary, over the next ten to fifteen years New York City and the United States will not experience any substantial increase in the number of the elderly, and particularly the frail elderly, that is persons over eighty-five. The large demographic shifts will occur after the year 2010, when the baby boom generation reaches retirement age. Nonetheless the steady upward drift in the number of the elderly will keep the question of how best to respond to their health and related needs in the foreground.

Responding to expenditures of over $400 million annually by New York City for care to Medicaid beneficiaries remaining in their own homes, the state legislature acted to cap the size of the program by capping the financial contribution of the state. With an average of about 50 hours per week of home care aides' services, the cost of preventing admissions to nursing homes comes high, circa $15,000 per person per year net of rent, food, and utilities.

To assess the prospect of a significant shift to home care, several interconnected questions need to be sorted out. As spokespersons for the elderly have stressed, other things being equal, most elderly prefer to remain at home rather than seek admission to a nursing home. But complicating factors of family, health, and money often intervene. It is much easier for a frail elderly person to remain at home if there are family members living in the same household or close by. The extent to which the homebound need assistance is a critical variable. One of the largest for-profit home health agencies has calculated that the upper bound is around four hours of daily assistance five days a week, or approximately 20 hours of externally provided care. Family or friends are expected to provide assistance over the weekend. Then there is the question of money. Is the elderly person using his own funds, or does he rely on public dollars? The range and quality of community services for the homebound and the availability of congregate housing are also important considerations.

Other factors that will influence the patterns of health care for the elderly in the remaining years of this century will be the expansion of DRG-based reimbursement, which will tend to shorten hospital stays and necessitate more intensive follow-up care at home for discharged patients; the extent to which the Medicare voucher gains acceptance and encourages large-scale enrollment of the elderly in HMOs and similar prepaid groups; improvements in medical technology and equipment that will ease the problems of caring for the severely disabled at home; and changing values among the elderly themselves that will affect decisions on heroic treatment and terminal care.

A middle-of-the-road forecast that does not pretend to assess definitively all of the foregoing factors suggests that there is likely to be a relative shift from inpatient to ambulatory and home care treatment settings; that if and when acute-care hospitals find themselves with excess capacity they are likely to convert some of their beds to rehabilitation and the care of the elderly; that more people will opt to die at home to avoid being subjected to extreme forms of medical or surgical intervention; and that the pressures on nursing home capacity will remain substantial for a variety of reasons, including the inability of many of the frail elderly to manage on their own.

The last forecast would be modified if medical research found techniques to slow, if not reverse, senile dementia and to assure bladder and bowel control among the elderly. It is unlikely that these breakthroughs will be realized within a single decade, but if they were, admissions to nursing homes would stabilize and might even decline.

The Hospitals' Training Role

So far we have concentrated on the changes that the different institutional settings within which health care has been provided—hospitals, physicians' offices, clinics, nursing homes, and home care—are likely to undergo in response to the preferences of patients, the expenditures of financiers, or alterations in the ways in which physicians and other health care providers shape their careers and their work.

We must now shift our focus to another critical dimension of the health care sector in New York City, that is, its role in the education and training of physicians both at the undergraduate and graduate level, which is a major function of the city's six academic health centers and their affiliated teaching hospitals. This educational function is directly and intimately linked to the provision of hospital and ambulatory care for a significant portion of the city's residents and plays a dominant role in the care provided the low-income population by the municipal hospitals, the Veterans Administration hospitals, and the inpatient and ambulatory services of the voluntary hospitals.

The disproportionate share of residency training. Health centers perform a disproportionate amount of the nation's residency training, roughly four times the city's share relative to its population. To a lesser degree, they also educate a differentially large number of undergraduate medical students, more than double New York's proportionate share. The vast scale of undergraduate and graduate instruction and training carried on in New York City requires us to consider the factors on the local, state, and national scenes that are likely to affect this particular dimension of the health care sector.

It is important to note that the assumption prevailing throughout the first three post-World War II decades—that the nation, New York State, and New York City would all profit from an enlarged output of physicians—is no longer conventional wisdom. The GMENAC report, published in 1980, presented an impressive body of data and analysis that questioned the perception of a continuing physician shortage. Admittedly, the leadership of U.S. medicine did not accept, surely not initially, the alternative finding of a prospective surplus. Despite the fact that New York City and New York State ranked among the highest in their ratios of physicians-to-populations, their political and professional leadership were also counted among skeptics. The State Board of Regents has persistently maintained that since many rural and low-income urban areas lack the number of private practitioners required to provide adequate care to their inhabitants, a policy of selective expansion in the training of physicians is necessary, surely desirable. Other state agencies, sensitive to the relatively small number of minorities in the medical profession and in the educational pipeline have also looked to an expansionary policy to correct these imbalances.

New York State, and in particular the New York metropolitan region, have also spawned a vociferous citizen lobby on behalf of state and federal action to facilitate the acceptance of a medical education abroad by their children who failed to gain admission to U.S. medical schools, despite the doubling of their capacity.

The borough of Queens has agitated for many years to become the site of a medical school, its leaders emphasizing repeatedly that Manhattan, Bronx, and Brooklyn each have at least one. In 1984 the state legislature finally transferred a modest sum, about $1.5 million, from the budget of the state university to that of the city university to encourage the latter to move ahead on planning for a medical school in Queens linked to the City University, of New York. Whether this authorization of funds will in fact bring the school into existence remains uncertain in the face of the state's disinclination to provide the bulk of the required funds; the determination of City College (located in Manhattan) not to relinquish the Sophie Davis School, which provides preclinical training for many minority students pursuing a medical education; and the preference of Downstate Medical Center to strengthen its linkages to its affiliates in Brooklyn rather than to expand to a Queens clinical campus.

Several other factors bearing on undergraduate enrollment should be added. SUNY-Downstate Medical School, which has the largest student body of any of the six schools in the city, has been advised by the accreditation authorities that it must improve its curriculum. The state of New York has been unwilling to invest more in Stony Brook, which remains a small school, far below original projections.

The State Health Commissioner also has recently acted to tighten the conditions under which U.S. citizens who study medicine in foreign schools may receive clerkships and staff appointments in hospitals in New York City.

In light of these conflicting forces and trends a cautionary view would suggest that the Queens medical school is likely to remain on the drawing board, possibly indefinitely. At the same time it is unlikely that there will be any cutback in the present level of undergraduate medical enrollment in the near term. A few years ago it was rumored that Albany would favor the elimination, through merger or relocation, of one of the private medical schools in New York City, but of late that has not been heard. And unless the state's budgetary condition were to worsen appreciably, it would appear that the Bundy money—state capitation aid to private institutions for the education of health care professionals—is likely to continue to be available.

Scope of residency training. The outlook for residency training is more complex. To begin with, much of the renown of the major academic health centers in New York City is directly linked to their long-term leadership in the field of graduate medical education. Some years ago when the state authorities, in an effort to reduce Medicaid reimbursement levels, placed a ceiling on the number of residents that the large teaching hospitals could include in their cost base for reimbursement, several of the leaders acted jointly to challenge this action in the courts, and won their case with the argument that the state officials had exceeded their authority in seeking to set an educational quota for these institutions.

The post-World War II decades have witnessed a shift in the staffing of the major teaching hospitals and this, in turn, has profoundly affected the manner in which different groups of patients are treated. The major teaching hospitals, which previously depended on attending physicians, are now dominated by full-time senior staff who admit and oversee the treatment of most private patients. However, they rely increasingly on residents and fellows to assist in much of the routine care, from preoperative testing to postoperative monitoring and support.

There is no way to draw a sharp demarcation between the educational experiences that the house staff is exposed to and the service functions they perform. Most informed observers believe that surely after the first year, the patient services provided by the house staff more than justifies the salaries they are paid and that their "pure" educational activities consume only a small proportion of their lengthy daily and weekly schedules.

The house staff is also responsible for much or most of the outpatient care provided in the emergency room and in the clinics and for the care of inpatients who are not admitted by a private physician, although a member of the full-time staff may assume formal responsibility to justify the hospital's claims for reimbursement under both Medicare B (professional services) and Medicare A (hospitalization).

In comparison with the major voluntary teaching hospitals, the residents' role in patient care is far greater in the municipal and the VA hospitals with which most teaching hospitals are affiliated. Since the early 1960s, when the affiliation program was introduced, the municipal hospitals have depended overwhelmingly on residents and fellows for providing ambulatory and inpatient care. True, the contracting teaching affiliate provides supervisory staff to assure that the prescribed diagnostic and therapeutic procedures are appropriate and are competently performed, but the great bulk of the care is provided by residents and the scope and quality of their supervision differs considerably among contractors and even among divisions and clinical departments under the control of the same contractor.

The relationship between the medical centers and the Veterans Administration hospitals has been relatively satisfactory these many years, largely as a result of the availability of substantial funding, which enabled the VA hospitals to maintain good support services as well as to pursue as impressive volume of in-house research and to support broad-based educational programs. More recently, funding from Washington has tightened and the VA hospitals are under increasing pressure to redirect their limited resources to expanding ambulatory care with corresponding economies in inpatient services that are the foundation for their cooperative residency programs. Research funding has also been cut back.

The primary affiliations of the academic health centers in New York City, however, have been with the much larger municipal hospital system. Three of the six medical schools—Downstate, New York University, and Einstein—depend in the first instance on a municipal hospital for most of their undergraduate and graduate clinical teaching. Mt. Sinai and Columbia are also affiliated with municipal hospitals, although these are less critical to their total teaching function. Only Cornell is without such an affiliation.

There have been, and continue to be, tensions between the contractors and the affiliates since the onset of the program in the early 1960s. The major difficulties have centered on deficiencies in the support services provided by the municipal hospitals, ranging from diagnostic equipment to nursing care. For its part, the city has repeatedly remonstrated that the contractors have been more concerned with providing acceptable training for their residents than with addressing the priority needs of the patients who seek care in the municipal hospitals and rotating staff to meet these needs. A quarter of a century after the inauguration of the affiliation program the conflicting interests of the two factions continue, with each round of negotiations seeking to narrow the gap.

It is unlikely that either party is in a position to withdraw from the contract, at least in the near term. If a radical reduction should occur in the number of inpatient days, conceivably the municipal hospitals could—in light of the easing of the physician market—recruit and retain an increasing number of full-time staff and thereby reduce their dependency on contractual agreements. But it is difficult to see how they could operate without a large complement of residents, and how these trainees could be attracted without the support of a major academic health center. Accordingly, the present uneasy alliance between the medical centers and the city's Health and Hospitals Commission is likely to persist for some years to come.

Financing. The future scale of residency training relates to the overarching issue of financing. It seems incredible, but is nonetheless a fact, that the vast expansion of graduate medical education during the past decades has come about in the absence of a generic financing mechanism. Aside from the nonmonetary transaction by which residents provided services in return for educational and training opportunities, most other costs incidental to their training were covered by reimbursements for patient care. Insurance and government accepted the costs of operating educational programs as a legitimate item in patient reimbursement.

Recently, challenges to this practice have begun to mount. The most important to have been raised thus far has been the unanimous recommendation of the Advisory Council to Social Security that a funding mechanism other than Medicare should be developed to support residency training. In initiating DRGs, Congress bypassed this issue by providing a pass-through for educational costs, but the secretary of HHS was directed to study this problem and come forward with specific recommendations as to the preferred ways of reimbursing hospitals for the additional costs of training residents.

The current pass-through provisions for DRGs that take into account not only direct educational outlays but also ancillary costs based on increased length of stay and greater intensity of care—both presumptively linked with residency training—have proved favorable to the academic health centers, but it is unlikely that Congress will continue them without change beyond the next few years. It remains unclear, however, what alternative approach will be acceptable to Congress, the states, and the private sector, each of which currently helps to underwrite graduate medical education and each of which will be under pressure to continue to support in one way or another this essential activity on which the medical care of the future is dependent.

The financing question is linked to the growing concern of many specialty societies about the number of residents who should be trained henceforth, the number of hospitals that may for economic or other reasons opt to reduce or terminate their training activities, and national and regional ratios of the number of U.S. medical graduates to the number of training slots. We are approaching a position where, for the first time, the two are in proximate balance, which means that any substantial reduction of the training programs could result in the failure of some graduates to gain admission into an approved program.

The outlook for residency training in New York City will be influenced by the interactions among several factors: the scale of the current programs; the dependency of the public hospitals (and also the voluntary hospitals) for the provision of patient care on the availability of large numbers of residents; the uncertainty of future financing from public and private sources for the higher hospitals costs associated with residency training, and the pressures arising within various specialty societies to scale back training programs. We cannot make even an educated guess as to the interactive effects of these discrete forces other than that, on balance, they point to a reduction over time in the scale and scope of residency training that will be carried out by the hospitals of New York City. If the payers for hospital care were to take radical action to decrease or eliminate their contributions for such training—an unlikely but not impossible eventuality—and if no satisfactory alternative were devised, the reduction could be substantial. The more likely development, however, will be modest cutbacks that over time could be absorbed without becoming a major threat to the provision of patient care or the training of tomorrow's physicians.

State Regulations

Currently, and for some time in the past, the state of New York has exercised substantial influence or control over hospital reimbursements, capital improvements, the regional distribution of services, and recently it has introduced an all-payer system to distribute the costs of care for the uninsured. There is no reason to believe that the state will withdraw from any of these activities and there is no reason to postulate that it will assume an even more prominent role in shaping the structure of the health care system in New York City and the remainder of the state. Moreover, indications from Washington point to a growing preference of the federal government to devolve more responsibility for the control of future outlays for health care onto the states. If we assume that such a policy will gain momentum—and this seems likely because of the difficulties of establishing national norms for the various states whose systems operate under quite different environmental conditions—we must anticipate a more active role for state officials in the reshaping of the city's health care system. A clue to the nature and intensity of the state's involvement is found in the pressure that it is exerting in response to the CON applications filed by the academic health centers. To both the Presbyterian Hospital and Mt. Sinai, the Commissioner of Health has indicated that approval was contingent upon a trade: the more these institutions were willing to undertake by way of assisting their neighboring communities—in the case of the Presbyterian, the establishment of a new community hospital in northern Manhattan, and in the case of Mt. Sinai, supporting North General Hospital in Harlem—the better their prospects for receiving approval. Similarly, Cornell, which is also seeking CON approval, has been urged to extend its existing ties with Jamaica Hospital in Queens.

The state has also indicated that it plans to step up its role in determining the location of expensive new services (for example,

MRI) with the aim of avoiding unnecessary, costly overcapacity and underutilization.

The legislature acted recently to strengthen the Health Systems Agencies, the planning bodies throughout the state, to get their feedback as to how finite capital funds should be allocated among the several regions so that priority needs may be met equitably. The federal government may act on the capital pass-through in the determination of Medicare reimbursement rates; thereafter the states are likely to have a clearer view of their future scope for action. But no matter what actions Congress takes regarding the capital pass-through, it is well nigh certain that New York state will continue to play a major role in shaping the directions of future hospital investments.

The remaining important arena for present and potential state action relates to all-payer arrangements to meet the costs of nonreimbursed care for the indigent. New York State has long been sensitive to this issue, and as early as 1970 enacted the Ghetto Medicine Program, which made special grants to help urban hospitals increase their services to the inner-city populations. In 1982 it received a waiver from the Department of Health and Human Services for Medicare reimbursement regulations to institute an all-payer system. This system imposes a levy on all hospitals to be contributed to a pool for distribution to those institutions that furnish large amounts of unrequited care, a levy that has continued even after the state opted out of the all-payer system.

Future Health Care in the City

In light of the many uncertainties that have been identified, it would be presumptuous to venture a definitive view of the future shape of the health care system in New York City with a prism focused on the years 1990–2000. However, a synthesis of the many discrete trends and possibilities that have been identified would be desirable if only to orient one to the longer future. We will venture the attempt, reemphasizing that the scenario contains many problematic factors; the uncertainty ratio is heightened when allowance is made for the interaction among the major elements. Despite these caveats, the effort may be justified.

· The relative role of hospital care within the health care system will decline in favor of greater reliance on ambulatory services, home care, and nursing home and hospice care.

· The major voluntary hospitals in New York City face a serious financial threat from DRG-based reimbursement because of their excessive lengths of stay. Even if the DRG approach should be radically modified or replaced, hospitals whose length of stay and per diem costs far exceed the average are certain to be under financial stress in a period of continuing price pressure.

· The combination of these two developments is likely to result, within the next ten years, in a shift from high occupancy rates to an excess of beds in most of the large hospitals.

· It is unlikely that the municipal hospital system, which experienced a substantial reduction of bed capacity in the preceding two decades, will shrink further through institutional closures in the period ahead. However, it is likely to reduce its total inpatient bed capacity as part of its capital rehabilitation program.

· The state of New York will continue to discourage the increase of nursing home capacity and will maintain a ceiling on the New York City home care program because of the serious implications of further expansion for state expenditures. The thrust of the state (as well as of the federal government and the voluntary sector) will be to strengthen community support efforts that will enable more of the frail elderly to be cared for in their own homes and communities. However, these constraining efforts may conflict with the reality of an expanded contingent of feeble elderly who will require institutional care, particularly if the restrictions on new capacity are maintained for the next five to ten years.

· The uncertainties regarding the future financing of graduate medical education point to prospective adjustments in the very large training programs in New York City, adjustments that are likely to result in reductions in training and in some cooperative arrangements among the major academic health centers for the conduct of high-cost, low-volume subspecialty programs. Such cooperative undertakings are not easy to negotiate and implement but they may be preferable to the complete elimination of selected programs. These developments are the more likely if individual specialty societies take the lead to cut back training programs and if the state throws its weight behind these reductions in the hope of moderating costs.

The more problematic issues involve the future of undergraduate enrollments, methods of financing the care of the poor, and the growth of new forms of health care delivery. We noted earlier that despite the long-time enthusiasm of Queens residents for a medical school within their borough and the recent transfer of state funds to the City University budget for planning purposes, serious questions remain about the feasibility of this long-term objective.

In fact, a trend to reduce undergraduate enrollments in the existing schools is not beyond the realm of possibility. New York University has already undertaken a small step in that direction. In a state that has long followed an expansionary policy, such a reduction will not be easy to effect, but it cannot be ruled out. If physicians in private practice experience a continuing decline in real income, they might persuade the legislature that cutbacks in the publicly supported schools would be desirable. This recommendation has been made to Downstate by the accrediting authority. The state could also cut back, even if it does not totally eliminate, capitation support for the private schools.

Since the major teaching hospitals and selected community hospitals provide a considerable amount of care to uninsured patients, and since most of them do not have the revenues to cover the costs of unreimbursed care, the state will confront the necessity of finding an alternative to the current all-payer system, which it has initiated by means of a Medicare waiver from HHS. If the waiver is terminated, the state will probably continue the all-payer system on its own initiative.

Perhaps the most problematic of future developments is the extent to which new forms of health delivery will emerge and succeed. HMOs do not appear to be poised for rapid growth, but the state, in cooperation with the city, may force the issue with regard to its Medicaid recipients. If the federal voucher for Medicare is made more attractive both to the beneficiaries and to the providers, this will also stimulate the growth of HMOs and other types of prepayment plans.

It is difficult to discern whether, on what scale, and how quickly the large teaching hospitals are likely to expand the scale and scope of their activities, from new ambulatory-care services for paying patients to rehabilitation and hospice care.

Even more difficult to assess is whether and in which areas new for-profit medical enterprises will succeed in entering the New York City market. The proprietary chains have given the city a wide berth in years past because they saw little opportunity for profits in an environment in which the state vigorously regulates reimbursement, licensing, and other facets of the system. Another deterrent is the prohibition by state law of the absentee ownership of hospitals. Since the state is likely to maintain tight control via CON, licensing, as well as rate setting, the odds are that a decade hence the for-profit institutions will still have a marginal role in New York City.

How Good a System Tomorrow?

The major issue is whether the present health care system is likely to perform as well or better in the future, both in meeting the health needs of the population and in encouraging the continued vitality of the system through its contributions to education and research. It is difficult to foresee a serious weakening in the major academic health centers. All but Downstate have sizable endowments, are linked to strong universities, and are closely affiliated with major voluntary hospitals. As for Downstate, it will probably continue to command substantial state and city resources.

As to the scale and quality of health care services that will be available to the citizenry as the century draws to a close, the prognosis must also be basically upbeat. There is no reason to believe that in combination, the large voluntary institutions, reinforced by the extensive municipal hospital system, should not be able to provide in the future, as they do at present and have in the past, a superior level of care to the more affluent population and an acceptable level to the poor and the near-poor. They should be able to meet this challenge despite a more constrained inflow of funds and necessary modifications in the locus of care. Only a collapse of leadership among the medical profession, the voluntary community, and city and state politicians— a highly unlikely eventuality—would place the system at serious risk. To the extent that the three groups deepen their understanding of the dynamics of change and develop more effective avenues of cooperation, the quality of care available to all should be improved. The above analysis, written five years ago, holds up more or less, except for the growing importance of AIDS patients and the tightening of bed capacity in both the municipal and voluntary hospitals, in part because of AIDS and in part because of the growing numbers of the elderly and the mentally ill who are being hospitalized.

· III ·

Medical Education, the Physician Supply, and Nursing

· 10 ·

The Reform of Medical Education

The quantity and quality of professional services available to the public depend, first, on the education and training of professionals and, second, on the ways in which a society organizes its delivery services. Education and service delivery are highly interdependent in the medical arena because of the dominant role of the physician, who has primary responsibility for diagnosis and therapy.

There is a consensus both within the United States and abroad that the quality of medical care available to most of the U.S. population is at an all-time high, the best in the world, and that the superior education and training of American physicians largely account for this strength. Why, then, should we recommend that medical education be reformed? The oversimplified answer is that the production, financing, and distribution of health care services in the United States are in the early stages of revolutionary change, and yet the numbers and types of physicians who will practice in the twenty-first century are being trained in response to the imperatives of an earlier era. The existing medical educational system is not providing the types of physicians who will be able to meet the changing health care needs of the public and to function in the newly emerging modes of health care delivery.

Neither we nor anybody else can pinpoint how this health care system will be structured and will operate in the decades ahead. However, we can chart the directions in which the new delivery system is evolving and can call attention to the changes in medical education required to keep the two in tandem.

Changes in Health Care Delivery

We are convinced of the need for medical education to reform itself because several major factors are altering—and will continue to alter—the delivery of health care services to the American people. The major payers for health care—government and corporations—are acting together to reduce their expenditures by encouraging various forms of prepaid and managed care arrangements. These will result in more and more physicians practicing as members of a team, often exposed to some financial risk because of payers' increasing preference for prepayment arrangements. There is intensified effort to substitute, wherever possible, ambulatory for inpatient treatment, to reduce costs. Such efforts, together with the parallel pressures to reduce the average length of hospital stay, will add to the excess capacity that increasingly characterizes the hospital sector and that presages the merger, conversion, and closure of many hospitals. Also on the grounds of economy and efficiency, payers and providers are intensifying efforts to make greater use of nonphysician health professionals, an increasing number of whom are seeking to bill patients directly. The American people have a growing interest in "wellness" programs; as a result, physicians need to counsel their patients on how they can best protect and enhance their health and well-being. At the same time the "gatekeeper" approach, in which the primary care physician determines under what conditions patients may be referred to specialists, is becoming more prevalent in managed care systems.

Not all changes are cost-related. For example, many patients insist on playing an active role in the decision making that affects alternative treatments; such physician/patient interaction will have consequences for therapeutic outcomes. New problems are also coming up with regard to the prolongation of life as a result of high-tech medical and surgical interventions. These issues require study not only by physicians but also by other professionals, such as lawyers and theologians, as well as by representatives of the public, to reassess the limits of modern medicine.

The composite effects of the foregoing changes on the delivery of health care point the directions in which physicians' mode of practice is likely to change in the decades ahead: from independent fee-for-service practice to membership in a prepaid group-practice arrangement based on a salary, often with some income risk sharing; from exercising one's independent judgment as to appropriate ways to diagnose and treat patients to being guided by group norms and protocols; from discretion to refer patients to specialists of one's own choosing to being limited to those on an approved list, with organizational pressures to keep referrals to a minimum; from being able to inform patients what they must do and anticipating that they will follow instructions to exploring their preferences and desires and reaching a joint decision before starting treatment; from having been looked upon as a highly respected professional who contributes greatly to the well-being of both patients and the community to being viewed increasingly as a professional who sells medical expertise in order to increase personal income; from being recognized as one possessing special knowledge and skill to becoming a practitioner in a demystified field whose members are increasingly being sued.

Changes within Medical Education

No matter how well medical education has responded in the past to the delivery of health care, it faces a major challenge in realigning itself with the new systems of health care delivery. It must also reconsider its goals and procedures as a consequence of new forces that are directly affecting the educational structure. At the end of this century the United States will have almost twice the number of physicians per 1,000 population that it had at midcentury. Since managed care systems use fewer physicians than fee-for-service practices use, the potential oversupply of physicians will be that much greater. There is a growing imbalance in the number of specialists and subspecialists[1] resulting from the new constraints that managed care systems are imposing on the referral of patients to specialists. Also, leaders in government, the profession, and the public recognize that remedial action, including radical reductions in the inflow of physicians trained abroad (foreign medical graduates or FMGs), is urgently required. In light of mounting evidence that further reductions loom ahead, young people are reassessing the attractiveness of medicine as a career, and their concerns go far beyond the probable decline in their earning capacity. Medical schools increasingly depend upon income derived from faculty practice plans (a pooling of group practice income with a portion going to the school and the department for their respective use). This points to reduced opportunities of faculty members to focus most of their attention on their educational and research activities.

Clearly, these major changes point to the need for broad reassessment and basic reforms. The urgency for such action is highlighted by the number of discrete and uncoordinated moves that threaten to weaken the existing structure of medical education without establishing a new, sound foundation to meet the challenges that lie ahead. At the beginning of the 1980s, the federal government terminated all direct support for medical schools, convinced that the long-standing shortage of physicians was over. In 1986 Congress acted to reduce the payments of Medicare for graduate medical education (GME). The federal government also has acted in recent years to reduce the flow of funding for student loan and grant programs. A few state legislatures have cut back their support for residency training, and many have moved to increase tuition in their medical schools, often steeply. Most private medical schools have raised their tuition to a level where many of the more prestigious institutions charge between $12,000 and $17,000 per year. In 1986, 82 percent of medical school graduates had incurred debts amounting on the average to $33,500; indebtedness levels of $50,000 or more are increasingly common. Several private medical schools have cut back their admissions. In Arkansas, for example, the legislature interdicted the plan of the faculty to reduce its class size. Clearly, such actions in no way constitute an adequate response on the part of medical education to the radical changes under way in the larger medical environment and in the practice of medicine.

We are convinced that the leaders of medical education—because they are the most knowledgeable about, and sensitive to, the long-term mission of the AHC—must take the initiative in proposing and carrying out the necessary and desirable reforms. In our opinion, developments are progressing at a rate that underscores the urgency with which medical educators must assess their options and responses. Unless they begin to coordinate their analyses and actions with universities and hospitals, insurers and government, the foundations of the U.S. medical educational system, which has served the public well over many decades, will be at serious risk.

Aware that each of our specific recommendations has been advanced before, we make no claim to originality. We believe, however, that we have provided the context and the rationale for early action if medical education is to prepare the number and types of physicians that the nation will need in the decades ahead.

The Rise of Third-Party Payers

Federal involvement. The Hill-Burton legislation, enacted in 1946, sought to improve access to care in rural areas by providing federal grants for the construction of rural hospitals. Urban teaching hospitals received federal and state funds to build and equip research facilities, including adding or remodeling patient care areas used for clinical research.

A vigorous new Veterans Administration addressed the problem of a sleepy, inefficient hospital system totally inadequate to care for the vastly increased, sicker, and more seriously disabled veteran population by establishing links between the major regional VA hospitals and neighboring medical schools. This arrangement gave medical schools access to new teaching beds and provided salaries for faculty assigned to the VA in return for recruiting physicians needed to care for the greatly enlarged numbers of hospitalized veterans.

Health insurance, as a fringe benefit for workers and their dependents, had expanded rapidly during World War II, when government authorities determined that insurance costs were approvable "in a reasonable amount" beyond wage rate increases under wage stabilization regulations. The postwar years saw the further rapid extension of health insurance.

Medicare and Medicaid. The enactment of Medicare and Medicaid in 1965 brought another massive infusion of money into the health care system. Whatever the initial concerns of the medical profession, these programs proved a bonanza for physicians and for most hospitals. Suddenly, there was public money to pay for the millions who had previously been medically indigent. Elderly persons, once forced to seek care in public hospitals or in the charity wards and outpatient departments of voluntary hospitals, now could pay for their care. This caused city and county hospitals to shrink and voluntary hospitals to change their approaches to the care of such patients. Large wards were replaced by private and semiprivate rooms. For a time it appeared that the two-tiered system of medical care, one for the affluent and one for the poor, soon would be eliminated.

Teaching hospitals in particular benefited from Medicare and Medicaid. Many beneficiaries of these programs had been admitted previously as charity patients in major teaching hospitals; now they could pay both for hospitalization and for the services of physicians. In addition, the federal government provided generous reimbursement for the direct and indirect costs of teaching, which quickly led to a doubling and tripling of residents' salaries; for the first time they received a reasonable stipend ($20,000). Physicians who supervised residency training likewise were paid for their services.

Postwar economics were such that the goal of almost every state-supported medical school was to have a new or reconstructed university hospital dedicated to teaching and research, supported by state appropriations, with unreimbursed patient care also covered by the state budget. Many states responded, lured by the promise of more and better physicians to practice within the state and the associated gain of a referral center for the seriously ill. Favorable tax laws, a concomitant of the booming postwar economy, and the efforts of professional fundraisers enabled many teaching hospitals to attract large amounts of philanthropic money.[2]

National Institutes of Health. Finally, a national strategy to improve the health of America emerged via the NIH external grant program. The decision to designate universities, medical schools, and affiliated teaching hospitals—instead of independent research centers—as the primary beneficiaries of NIH grants was fateful for medical education. The mission of NIH was, and is, to promote basic and applied biomedical research that directly or indirectly improves the health of the nation. Because of congressional mandates, NIH focused on categorical diseases: cancer, heart disease, and so on. The NIH grant mechanism was never intended to provide direct support for medical education. But the NIH design had a powerful and reinforcing influence on medical school departments that become increasingly focused on the teaching and practice of specialized medicine. Inasmuch as the institutes of NIH were categorically organized, it is not surprising that NIH training programs for clinical specialties were directed to the subspecialties of medicine such as cardiology or gastroenterology.

Encouraged to believe that more money would lead to earlier cures of such dread afflictions as cancer, heart disease, and stroke, Congress's appropriations increased by about 18 percent per annum (in inflation-free dollars) between 1950 and 1965. In response, medical schools and clinical residency programs aligned and realigned their clinical and subspecialty divisions and their research training programs, so that they were better positioned to attract more of the enlarged flow of federal dollars. Soon, NIH support not only reflected but also accelerated the trend to specialization in U.S. medicine.

Expansion of Medical Schools and Academic Medicine

Rapid economic growth and the expectation that it would continue facilitated the expansion of medical schools, fueled by the widespread perception of a serious shortage of physicians. Evidence in support of this belief included the long waiting periods before patients with nonemergency conditions could consult a physician and the difficulties experienced by small towns and rural America in recruiting young physicians to replace practitioners who were retiring or who had died. (Actually, the rural shortage reflected in part the reluctance of newly trained physicians to practice in areas with limited hospital facilities.) The misperception of serious shortages was aggravated by the trend from general practice toward specialization and the growing maldistribution of physicians.

By the mid-1960s Congress passed a series of health manpower bills that supported the construction of new medical schools and the expansion of class size in existing schools. The result was an increase in the number of medical schools from 88 in 1964–65 to 127 in 1986–87, and a doubling in the size of the graduating class, from 7,409 to 15,872 during the same time span.

Academic medicine responded to congressional action in part because it, too, perceived a shortage, but also because of the financial payoff attached to enlarging their classes—namely, a capitation allowance for each enrolled student and an additional allowance for each graduate. The tightening of NIH support made the new capitation provisions particularly attractive, because the added funds became available to the dean to use for schoolwide, rather than departmental, priorities.

The impact of these developments on medical education was profound. Over the twenty-year period from 1946 to 1965, academic medicine was totally reshaped. Only the medical school curriculum, despite the efforts of some thoughtful reformers, remained relatively unchanged. Beginning in 1948, the infusion of NIH funds permitted the rapid expansion of the full-time faculty in both clinical and preclinical (basic science) departments. It is important to note that the increase in faculty during the period 1950–1986 was directly linked to research, research training, and the development of subspecialty divisions within the specialties. Also during the twenty-year period following World War II, clinical departments in teaching hospitals assumed their present shape, with large subspecialty divisions dominating most aspects of departmental activity. Although most medical schools continued to use part-time faculty for clinical teaching, the importance of part-timers waned as the size and power of the full-time faculty increased.

Rise of the academic health center. During this initial period, the AHC—defined as a medical school, one or more primary teaching hospitals, one or more other health professional schools such as a nursing school or dental school, often a VA hospital, and one or more affiliated community hospitals with residency programs—evolved and matured. While no two AHCs are alike, the new nomenclature aptly defines the conglomerate organization that replaced the relatively simple medical school structure of earlier times.

By 1966 most of the important changes in academic health centers were in place, although many of their consequences had not yet become fully manifest. In that year, the future of academic medicine appeared to be boundless. NIH funding for research and research training appeared to be assured; the budget of NIH had been increased sufficiently each year to fund new investigators without cutting off those with previous support. No great financial sacrifice was required of researchers opting for academic careers; applications to medical school were up and the quality of applicants was high; and Medicare and Medicaid gave promise that teaching hospitals would be much better supported than in the past.

By 1966 AHCs had achieved a position of dominance, not only because of their educational and research roles, but also because they provided the most advanced medical care. The primary teaching hospitals of the AHCs, whether university-owned or not, became models for large community hospitals that wanted to be in the vanguard of subspecialty medicine. Over time the AHCs came to control almost all residency training, since few residency programs dependent on graduates of U.S. medical schools survived outside of hospitals affiliated with AHCs. This meant that the AHCs, together with the various specialty boards and residency review committees, determined the scale and scope of specialty training as well as the specialty distribution of physicians.

But rapid expansion does not assure continuing stability, and by the late 1960s a reduction in the rate of increase of the NIH budget was the first signal that there might be trouble ahead. The tightening of Medicare reimbursement was a second signal. Other, equally serious problems began to emerge.

Problems of AHCs. It is an article of faith among most academic physicians that the AHC is (or at least should be) an integral part of the university. The deans of health professional schools other than medicine believe that their schools belong to a partnership of equals within the AHC structure. Both are ideals, and both are remote from reality. Governance varies among AHCs, but whatever their formal structure, power has always been with the heads of the clinical departments and the heads of the divisions since they control most of the funding. The result is a confederation of semiautonomous baronies.

Liberal funding for research and research training only reinforced the attitudes and behavior of preclinical and clinical faculty members, both having become more interested in research than in the education of medical students. The so-called preclinical disciplines or basic sciences—which for years have been regarded as applied, even cookbook, sciences—became in the postwar era the source of some of the most exciting advances in molecular and cell biology as well as in immunology. Graduate students were attracted to these departments because financial support was available and because the future of academic medicine held great promise.

It should be no surprise that a research-oriented preclinical faculty would become more engaged in the education of graduate students dedicated to the preclinical disciplines than in the training of medical students who, except for the unusually able few enrolled in joint M.D.-Ph.D. programs, had only a transient interest in their respective fields. Of course, some preclinical faculty members remained devoted to the education of medical students. But the criteria used in the recruitment of new faculty members tended to emphasize research abilities rather than a commitment to teaching, particularly since junior faculty members were expected to compete for their own research funding, which often was used to cover a portion of their salaries.

The change in the teaching interests of the clinical faculty was, if anything, even more dramatic. Prior to World War II, residency programs in the major medical schools were dedicated more to the training of young physicians for academic medicine than for specialty practice, and board certification following residency training was considered less important than years of research experience in a distinguished laboratory. There were few formal training programs in the medical subspecialties, and the relatively small full-time clinical faculty took seriously its commitment to the teaching of medical students. Many part-time voluntary faculty members were equally devoted to teaching undergraduates.

While preparing physicians for careers in academic medicine remained an important goal, most clinical departments recognized that the majority of their residents and fellows would become practitioners rather than investigators. It may seem paradoxical that clinical departments were more interested in training physicians for academic medicine before World War II than after World War II (a period characterized by liberal support for research training), but it is important to recall that before World War II, most medical school graduates took only one year of internship in a community hospital. Hence the number seeking residency training in academic departments was both smaller and more selective.

Medical school curriculum. Despite the striking changes in patterns of physician education and practice, little change has occurred in the structure of the medical school curriculum since 1910. Approximately two years are still devoted to basic sciences and the same amount of time to clinical medicine. The basic medical science departments are preserved in much the same disciplinary array as in earlier times, even though everyone recognizes that a modern molecular cell biologist can be equally at home in a university department of biology, biochemistry, microbiology, physiology, or pharmacology.

Medical educators rationalize the long-standing demarcation in clinical education—undergraduate and graduate—as "general education" and "specialized training." Their rationale ignores the fact, however, that often the same clinical educators teach both medical students and housestaff (residents), that medical students spend far more time with housestaff than with the clinical faculty, and that each clinical discipline teaches what it knows best, namely, specialized medical knowledge. Moreover, by the 1980s few academic physicians were qualified to teach medicine as a general discipline.

The artificial separation of undergraduate and graduate clinical education has to do mostly with jurisdiction. Medical schools control the education of medical students but not residency training. Members of the medical school's clinical faculty, together with the national specialty boards and residency review committees, which they dominate, control residency and fellowship training, but they exercise their authority outside the jurisdiction of the medical school and the university.

Clinical departments have good reasons for seeking to maintain this separation of powers. Each clinical department sets the curriculum for its own residency and fellowship training in accordance with the ground rules established by the national accrediting bodies. It does not have to consult with any other department or with the dean. Each clinical department also is able to compete nationally for the best residency candidates and has no special obligation toward the graduate training of its own medical school graduates. Clinical departments cherish these privileges and freedoms, and are loath to share them.

One could assume that the enormous size of medical school faculties, with a ratio of faculty members to medical students of approximately one to one, would lead to an intimate tutorial-like environment. Yet medical faculties are probably more remote from their students than are most college and university faculties, with their far smaller ratios of faculty to students. It is because the huge faculty reflects the pervasive emphasis on research, graduate medical education, and specialty practice, not the education of medical students.

Some attempts have been made to teach basic medical sciences in an integrated fashion, as in the Case Western Reserve experiment of the early 1950s. The principal change in the preclinical curriculum, however, has been the teaching of pathophysiology. Here the pathology of disease is taught in terms of the deepened understanding of physiology and biochemistry and, more recently, cell and molecular biology. The irony is that subspecialists in the clinical departments often are better equipped to teach pathophysiology than are most of their basic science colleagues.

Another significant change in the preclinical years has been the deemphasis of laboratory experience, in no small measure a reflection of the increasing cost and complexity of modern apparatus. One of the most constructive reforms attributed to Flexner in his guide to modernizing medical education was "learning by doing," which included carrying out experiments in the course of learning the rudiments of the basic medical sciences. Today, the time spent in the laboratory during the first two years of medical school has declined as the time spent listening to lectures has increased.

Sources of funding. As NIH funding plateaued and competition for research grants intensified, faculty practice plans replaced the federal government as the major source of revenue for U.S. medical schools. Departments differed in their ability to generate income, with the surgical subspecialties the largest earners and departments of pediatrics the smallest. Overall, an impressive surplus developed above and beyond the sums needed to pay the salaries of the full-time clinical faculty. The increase in the size of clinical faculties from 1950 to 1986 came in two waves—one in the 1960s associated with liberal research funding, the other in the 1970s related to the increasing importance of faculty practice plans. Today, concerns about the funding of medical education have been intensified by the potential plateauing of faculty practice income—the largest source of medical school income—as the practice of medicine becomes more competitive and pressures for cost containment increase.

Foreign medical graduates. Compounding the supply and financing problems is the large number of FMGs who have entered this country since World War II—primarily graduates of schools in Southeast Asia and Latin America. More recently, large numbers of American citizens who had been denied admission to medical schools in this country have enrolled in foreign medical schools—in Mexico, the Caribbean, and Europe. At the end of 1985, 118,875 FMGs were in active practice, representing 21.5 percent of all active physicians. Many were recruited originally to fill residency positions in community hospitals and public hospitals during the years of rapid growth.

In summary, during the years after World War II medical schools were absorbed into the vast conglomerates of AHCs. Although conceived as extensions of universities, these AHCs became increasingly detached from their parent university because of their concern with the provision of patient services. The dependence of AHCs on a variety of outside funding sources has led them to increase faculty size in response to their needs for research, for graduate medical education, and for patient care rather than for the teaching of medical students. Accompanying this growth of the AHC, the education of the physician became much longer and more expensive, as residency and fellowship training became, if not universal, widespread. Postgraduate education lasting three to seven years became a far more important part of clinical education that the clinical experience acquired in medical school. Medical faculties grew for reasons that had little to do with the education of medical students and much to do with the flow of research dollars, yet there was very little change in the structure of the medical school curriculum: it continued to reflect its developers' commitment to a balance between preclinical and clinical education. The modern U.S. medical school is now responsible for half, or less than half, of the education of the physician (the rest consists of residency and fellowship programs), and each half is under a different system of oversight and control. The result is serious discontinuity between the two parts of the educational experience.

More and more physicians enter practice each year, partly as the result of an expansion in the size and number of American medical schools and partly as the result of a continuing influx of FMGs. The rapid growth continues despite GMENAC's predictions of surplus; because of the nature of graduate medical education, specialists account for the major portion of the surplus. The greatly increased medical school capacity after the mid-1960s, aided and abetted by civil rights efforts and the availability of federal dollars, created a favorable environment for increasing the number of minority applicants who were admitted. The much enlarged output of physicians resulted in a flow of many newly trained specialists into smaller communities, which improved the medical care available to these populations.

Economics and public policy, rather than educational philosophy, have thus influenced the structure and content of medical education since 1964, and graduate medical education has taken precedence over the teaching of medical students in terms of both faculty interest and emphasis. Despite periodic efforts at reform, the dominant medical school curriculum continues to rely heavily on lectures to pack more and more technical information into students during their preclinical years. Clinical teaching is oriented to the specialties and subspecialties of medicine and assumes that all students will eventually specialize and will have a minimum of three or more years of clinical training after receiving the medical degree.

Challenges to Medical Education

One reason for the failure of medical educators to adapt to the realities of the 1980s has been the rigidity of the established systems that is sharply demarcated by four years of college, four years of medical school, and three to seven years of graduate medical education. The inflexibility of this structure has made it almost impossible to introduce new subjects into an already overcrowded medical school curriculum, which, in part, reflects redundancies between college science and medical school science, as well as between clinical experience in the last two years of medical school and clinical experience during the three to seven years of graduate medical education. As a result of this rigidity, medical schools no longer have a clear-cut goal for undergraduate medical education. Is it to prepare students for the specialty practice of medicine, or for general practice, and if the latter, to what purpose and end?

Financial pressures. Genuine efforts to alter the system are urgently needed if only because of the steadily increasing financial pressures on most medical students and medical schools. Chief among these pressures are student indebtedness and the changes in reimbursement for graduate medical education. Concerns about indebtedness definitely have reduced the number of medical school applicants from lower socioeconomic groups and have influenced the choice of specialty among graduates. Regarding reimbursement, it is now generally acknowledged that graduate medical education, not the education of medical students, accounts for the larger portion of the educational costs of future physicians. Since the mid-1980s both the federal government and other third-party payers have signaled their intent to cut back on their support for graduate medical education. In the past, specialty boards and residency review committees were able to set the standards and dictate the length of time that residents were required to spend in training, but these organizations have had no fiscal responsibility for the programs that they govern. In the face of growing surpluses of physicians and specialists, third-party payers have begun to reduce the level of their expenditures for graduate medical education via patient care reimbursement.

Declining applicant pool. Substantive issues beyond financial changes also deserve attention. There has been a striking decline in the pool of well-prepared college students applying to medical schools, a decline that can be traced back to the mid-1970s. For instance, in 1975, 32,515 men applied to medical school; in 1986 the figure had dropped to 20,056. Had it not been for the large and increasing pool of well-prepared women applicants, U.S. medical schools would have been unable to maintain the quality of their entering classes. Evidence now points to a leveling off in the number of female applicants and a continuing decline in male applicants during the remaining years of this decade and possibly into the 1990s. There also is evidence that the growing anxieties and disgruntlement expressed by many members of the profession are influencing the career choices of many superior college students, discouraging them from applying to medical school.

In light of these trends, it surely is time to reassess the mission of undergraduate medical education. In one sense, it is still the same: to meet societal needs by preparing competent physicians in the numbers and for the specialties that the American population will require. In another sense, it is vastly different, considering the rapidly changing nature of our medical care system and the enormous additions to medical knowledge during this century. In 1910, medical school graduates were ready for practice after one year of internship; in 1987, they are not. In 1910, there was a severe limit to what physicians were able to do. Today, the knowledge base, the technology of medicine, and physician competence have increased exponentially.

What, in the 1980s, should a medical school graduate be prepared to do? Although experts differ in their views, many would agree that the majority of graduates should be prepared to provide primary care without further training, a small percentage should continue to train for careers in research and teaching, and a larger percentage should complete training in one or another of the specialties of medicine.

Training requirements. Whether graduates plan to become primary care physicians, teachers, or specialists, they will need to hone problem-solving abilities and understand the role of uncertainty in medical decision making; to gain access to, and to use effectively, the ever-larger pool of medical information, which means acquiring computer literacy; to talk to patients, and even more important, learn to listen; to develop a greater understanding of the role of the physician in today's society; to be sensitive to the moral and ethical issues that affect responsibilities toward medical care system; to have the technical competence to practice medicine; and to continue training to keep abreast of the expanding knowledge base and the technology of medicine.

Redefining the Mission of Medical Schools

Medical schools need to reaffirm their primary mission. The country needs more primary care physicians and fewer specialists. The American Medical Association, the Association of American Medical Colleges, the specialty boards, and the residency review committees would benefit by becoming more responsive to the needs of the general public and by devolving some of their authority and responsibility to medical school faculties. We believe that it would be in the interest of all parties to consider and initiate major reforms while there is still time for orderly change.

Duration of medical training. We believe it is feasible to reduce significantly the time it takes to prepare a primary care physician (or specialist) without sacrificing quality. Much has been written about the importance of general education and a broad college experience. Efforts to educate more humane physicians through changed requirements favoring greater exposure to the liberal arts and social sciences over exclusive attention to the natural sciences are important. While we support general education, we would point out that most college students start to specialize in some discipline by the end of their sophomore year, with a significant number selecting a major even earlier. Students at Oxford or Cambridge planning to enter medicine complete the first one-and-one-half years of medical school before they receive their bachelor of arts degree in physiology. Few would claim that they are poorly educated. For good students, therefore, the problem appears to be more a question of turf than of education. There are numerous examples of successful programs that have bridged the college experience and the first two years of medical school. Many students are fully qualified to enter medical school at the end of their third year of college, a practice that was widespread before World War II and that has had its emulators in recent decades.

Such a plan, however, is feasible only for the student who is certain of a career track and has enrolled in a university that has a medical school. It does not help the student in a liberal arts college. In this instance the medical school must take the initiative and admit the student after three years of college, either as a regular medical student or with deferred admission, based on the student's ability to take the equivalent of the first year of medical school at the liberal arts college, perhaps enrolling for summer courses at another institution. If the student were given deferred admission in the spring of the junior year, there would be two summers in which to take courses not offered at the liberal arts college.

Four consecutive years of clinical training (the last two years of medical school and two years of graduate medical education), interspersed with some course work, would be ample for training the general internist, the general pediatrician, and the family physician. For one thing, much of the fourth-year medical student's time currently is spent on elective courses outside the framework of a coherent educational plan. During this year, the student devotes an inordinate amount of time, effort, and money applying for residency training, a process that involves visits to numerous teaching hospitals around the country. Second, if the clinical faculty had an opportunity to plan four years of clinical experience rather than two, more effective use could be made of the time through the design of a more rational curriculum. The argument may be raised that students profit by going to different institutions for residency training and that a six-year integrated program would be unduly restrictive. This criticism could be met if selected medical schools formed consortia that were willing to exchange students for parts of their undergraduate or graduate experience.

What about those who plan to specialize in a surgical field, radiology, psychiatry, or some other specialty? Such individuals should begin to specialize after three years of clinical training rather than four, with their prior clinical training accepted as the first year of their residency requirement. This would eliminate at least one year from the time required for board certification in a specialty.

Curriculum revision. The planning of the new curriculum would need to be done in cooperation with the appropriate specialty boards and would require the participation of all clinical departments. Clearly, not every student would take the same clinical curriculum; training for a surgical career would differ from the curriculum designed for an internist or pediatrician. Most students have a good idea of their clinical interests by the end of their first clinical year; indeed, in the present system, they must select the specialty they wish to enter soon after their first clinical year, since applications for residencies are made at the start of the second clinical year. Therefore, there would be no difficulty after the first clinical year in distinguishing among students wishing to enter general medicine, surgery, radiology, pediatrics, and so on. Many would know even earlier.

The first clinical year would require little change, since in most medical schools it is devoted to intensive exposure to the major specialties of medicine. To be sure, there is growing concern about the appropriateness of the teaching environment in the tertiary care hospital, particularly now that length of patient stay has been shortened. However, that is a generic problem that needs to be solved regardless of the changes suggested here. What could be designed in a more rational fashion is the educational experience that follows the first clinical year.

Most educators would agree that the future surgeon needs more exposure to the medical specialties that he or she is likely to receive now. Similarly, the future general internist, general pediatrician, or family physician needs greater familiarity with surgical problems, including those common to the urologist and orthopedist, than such a generalist is likely to have now. Both surgical and medical specialists also would benefit from well-designed clerkships in psychiatry, since all physicians ultimately care for many individuals with emotional as well as physical problems. The point is that designing the curriculum for each specialist in a four-year block would provide needed clinical experiences outside of the chosen specialty.

Clinical training. Medical schools also need to reexamine the setting for the clinical teaching of medical students, since tertiary care hospitals have become increasingly inappropriate sites to carry on the larger part of their clinical training. Many patients are being worked up before admission; diagnosis-related groups have shortened the number of days that patients spend in the hospital; and much of the treatment that once went on in the hospital is now performed in ambulatory settings. Medical schools need to identify ambulatory settings in which to carry out much of their teaching function. Identifying alternatives to inpatient sites as well as structuring and supervising such clinical training present many difficulties. Even more difficult will be the shift of funds that will be required to cover the educational costs in ambulatory sites in an increasingly competitive practice environment.

AHCs were formed in the belief that there was a congruence in mission between the medical school and its principal teaching hospital. This may no longer be true, as the teaching hospital needs to maintain and strengthen its highly specialized tertiary care services, and the medical school is forced to establish new ties with groups whose work is centered in ambulatory care settings. Both the teaching hospital and the medical school have important missions, but they are not identical. It is important for each to recognize that its interests do not always coincide with those of the other. The medical school should remain an integral part of the university, but the major teaching hospital should be an autonomous institution outside the governance of the university. Hospital and medical school can then cooperate when it is mutually beneficial, but also pursue their separate ways when that is desirable.

Under this approach, the medical school could, for example, have a much smaller full-time faculty whose clinical members would be dedicated to the education of medical students. This core faculty, paid out of the budget of the medical school or university, would have the full responsibility for designing both the basic science and clinical portions of medical education. The members of the clinical faculty would call on physicians working in the affiliated teaching hospitals and ambulatory care settings for assistance and support and would have, with the dean's consent, the authority to contract with part-time teachers.

With this change in the structure of medical schools, the students would save one year of tuition at the interface between college and medical school. They would pay full tuition during the first two years in medical school and for the first full clinical year; pay possibly one-half tuition for the second clinical year, recognizing they would be providing some service to patients; pay no tuition during the third year, possibly receiving a partial stipend; and receive a full stipend during the fourth clinical year.

Financial support. Medical education also faces the need to realign functions and financial support. In the future, the dean's freedom to commingle funds for education, research, and patient care will be restricted further, and medical schools and teaching hospitals must reexamine, while they still have time, their faculty needs in each of these areas. Thus it is essential to have a core full-time faculty whose primary function is integrating the collegiate-preclinical science interface, as well as planning the clinical curriculum up to the first certification of primary care specialists.

Teaching hospitals should not, nor will they, turn their backs on multispecialty group practices supported by patient care income, whose primary educational concern is specialty training.

But there should be a clear understanding that such faculty members, whether designated full time or part time, are not the direct financial responsibility of the medical school. It will be necessary to enlist the help of such faculty members in teaching medical students, particularly in the departments of medicine, pediatrics, obstetrics, and psychiatry. Similarly, since the assistance of physicians practicing in ambulatory care settings not associated with the primary teaching hospital will be needed, faculty appointments may be appropriate for some or all of them. The medical school will have to contribute to these teaching costs, but, again, with the understanding that the salary for such individuals does not come primarily from the budget of the medical school. The enormous size of current faculties has less to do with the teaching of medical students than with the provision of patient care, specialty training, and research.

Role of biomedical research. We recognize and applaud the enormous contribution that the biomedical research community has made to the science and technology of medicine and would welcome the day when NIH support could be further increased, since there are many more strong research proposals than available funds. We do not accept, however, the proposition that research, patient care, and teaching are inseparable, or that the quality of education will be diminished greatly if it is carried out in an environment in which research is not the dominant activity. Some first-rate researchers are very good teachers, and some are not. There is often no close correlation between those who are the best teachers and those who are the best investigators. And there certainly is none between the best researchers and the best practitioners of medicine. What is needed is not the continuation of an artificial commingling of functions, but the recognition that serious teaching is a difficult and demanding activity, and that two lectures a year to a large medical school class do not qualify as serious teaching.

The great diversity among AHCs is partly reflected in the quantity and quality of research they perform. That 16 percent of AHCs receive 50 percent of NIH funding suggests the variations in research effort. It is our view that research funding is likely to become more, rather than less, competitive, and that the most successful investigators will be those who pursue research as their primary activity. This does not mean that the supply of able teachers necessarily will be reduced, but only that good teaching must be recognized as a primary activity in its own right—and be appropriately rewarded. Not all AHCs must aspire to strong research programs to have able teachers on their faculty, any more than research-intensive AHCs can rely on superior investigators to assure superior teaching. Nevertheless, a strong research environment will enhance the productivity of the educational experience.

Continuing Issues

Because of the commingling of funds, no one knows just what it costs to educate a medical student to first certification. New efforts should be made to ascertain these costs. The need for close supervision during the early clinical years suggests that the costs will prove to be considerable, but it is highly unlikely that they will equal or even approximate the frequently cited estimate of $50,000 per year.

More to the point, who should pay? The mission of NIH is not to support medical education, except insofar as it supports the training of future investigators, as in M.D.-Ph.D. programs. Faculty practice plans, now the major source of support for medical schools, are inappropriate, since they thrive on highly specialized, high-tech procedures that have very little to do with the education of medical students. Some support can come from increased tuition, but tuition cannot be relied upon as a major source of funding in view of the current need to extend loans to such a large part of the student body both in private and in public institutions. Even in the wealthiest schools, endowment income is insufficient. State schools traditionally have looked to their legislatures for additional support, but the outlook is less favorable now that the country is seen to face an oversupply of physicians. And the same is true for states that provide partial support for private medical schools. As noted earlier, direct support of medical education by the federal government has been discontinued, and there is no prospect, in light of the predicted surplus of physicians, that it will be reinstituted. Third-party payers are seeking to reduce, if not withdraw totally, the indirect support they currently provide for medical education via payments for patient care. Any serious effort to reform medical education must confront this critical need to unbundle educational costs and address them directly.

The number of medical school applicants has dropped from a peak of over 42,000 in 1975–1977 to approximately 31,300 in 1986–87, and the decline is likely to continue, if not accelerate. The size of the entering class peaked at 17,320 in 1981–82 and has decreased since then some 0.6 percent a year to 16,779 in 1986–87. The decline began even before there was a drop-off in the cohort of twenty-two-year-olds in the population. A medical career no longer appears as attractive to able college students. Judging by test scores and grade point averages, there has been no significant deterioration as yet in the overall quality of applicants, but some state schools that exclusively or primarily admit only in-state residents have found it increasingly difficult to maintain their previous selection criteria.[3]

Nothing on the horizon suggests that the decline in medical school applicants will reverse itself, nor does it appear that the projected surplus of physicians has been overestimated. Thus we conclude that the capacity of the nation's medical schools should be reduced drastically. Probably the best way to achieve these reductions would be to reverse what was done to achieve the increase. The weakest schools should be closed; some of these would be schools that were established recently in response to the presumed physician shortage. States with more than one medical school should consider a reduction in their number, possibly through consolidation. Similarly, states with both public and private medical schools should explore whether one or more mergers could be achieved. Finally, all schools should consider a reduction in class size once the quality of their applicant pool begins to slip to a point at which they have to lower their standards of admission to maintain their current class size.

As far as reducing the inflow of FMGs, recent reforms are in the right direction. Only those FMGs who meet the test scores of U.S. graduates should be accepted for residency training; Medicare funding for residency training for those who do not pass should be withdrawn.

Changes in the Health Care System

Drop in hospital use. Hospital utilization rates will continue to drop. Moreover, admissions have begun to decline with an accelerated decline in the average length-of-stay. Even conservative tertiary care hospitals estimate that they are able to perform about 30 percent of their surgical load in an ambulatory setting, and well-managed community hospitals that conduct teaching programs believe that a decade from now ambulatory surgery may approach 70 percent. Even if the current trend stops short of the most extreme projections, many surgical residents now encounter a patient for the first time under anesthesia in the operating room, and, because of increasingly early discharge, residents have little opportunity to follow the patient during recovery.

This trend toward reduced reliance on inpatient care and abbreviated hospital stays greatly modifies the principal learning environment for residents and, to a lesser degree, undergraduate medical students. With workup and follow-up increasingly being undertaken outside the hospital, and with many conditions being treated from start to finish in an ambulatory setting, medical educators face radical adjustments in their mode of teaching if their students are to be exposed to a broad range of clinical problems.

Increase in ambulatory care. As the hospital inpatient service becomes less favorable for the teaching of residents, more ambulatory care sites will be available where a steady flow of patients is diagnosed and treated in a group-practice setting. With a little ingenuity, medical education could shift a good part of its clinical teaching from inpatient to ambulatory care settings. But the shift will not be easy. One reason is that the current principal source of financing for graduate medical education is patient care reimbursement derived from Medicare and insurance. It would take considerable goodwill and careful planning by payers and providers to have part of the present funding for graduate medical education transferred from hospital to ambulatory care sites.

Further, the new ambulatory sites are operating in an increasingly competitive environment where the efficient and effective processing of large numbers of patients is a *sine qua non* for survival and growth. The presence of students, particularly undergraduates but also first-year residents, participating in patient care activities is certain to retard "productivity." This is not an insuperable obstacle to the teaching of students and residents in ambulatory settings, but it would require new funding sources to cover the additional costs. At present, such sources do not exist, and in an environment in which payers are seeking to reduce, not increase, their subsidy to medical education, developing new funding sources will not prove easy.

A reduction in the need for training opportunities in the future may help. If the number of admissions to U.S. medical schools and the number of FMGs accepted into residency training are cut back, and if there is a reversal in the trend from subspecialty training in favor of primary care, some of the present funding might be shifted more easily to help finance training in ambulatory sites. Under these circumstances, the residency review committees are well-positioned to act aggressively to reduce the number and size of the current training programs. There will be resistance from directors of training as well as from the administrators and boards of trustees of community hospitals that have long sponsored training programs. However, the reduction of governmental support for graduate medical education, simultaneously with the improved prospects of hospitals to hire physicians for part- or full-time work at salaries competitive with those of residents, should temper the opposition. We do not contend that every community or governmental hospital that now depends heavily on residents to cover its patient load will find the shift to alternative staffing easy; we do suggest that in time it probably can be accomplished without adverse effects for patient care.

Growth of prepaid health care. The growth of prepayment systems reinforces the desirability of restricting both the total numbers of physicians who will be trained and the numbers trained in the medical and surgical subspecialties. In 1987 the average ratio of physicians per 100,000 population was in the 220–230 range for the United States as a whole, up from 140 in the early years after World War II. Current estimates put the ratio at 240 by the end of this decade and around 270–280 by the turn of the century. Prepayment plans that deliver medical care to designated population groups employ a ratio of about 110 physicians per 100,000 enrollees, roughly half the present national average. Alvin Tarlov, president of the Henry J. Kaiser Family Foundation and former chair of GMENAC, noted that the large surplus forecast by the committee in 1980 will be considerably larger as a result of the rapid growth of prepayment plans.[4] The parallel growth of managed care plans foreshadows a marked decline in referrals to specialists. Patients in these plans, unlike those in fee-for-service arrangements, are not free to consult a specialist as they wish. If the plan is expected to cover the cost of the consultation, patients may see a specialist only when the visit is authorized by their primary care physician.

Declining referrals. The major teaching hospital affiliates of the AHCs also are being affected by the reluctance of the staffs of outlying hospitals, principally those in the suburbs, to continue to refer a wide range of cases. Over the years, the AHCs had trained their own competition, and as patient loads decline, many suburban physicians and hospitals tend to retain all the cases they feel competent to treat.

There also will be continued proliferation of preferred provider arrangements. These plans do not readily facilitate the admission of patients to teaching institutions whose costs are often far above those of the average hospital. The heart of PPAs' approach is to obtain health care at the lowest cost by using their consolidated purchasing power in a market with excess hospital beds and specialists. AHCs have begun to reposition themselves by downsizing, strengthening their referral networks by establishing their own HMOs, or entering into arrangements with existing HMOs or PPAs (particularly for patients requiring tertiary care), and by old or new linkages with smaller hospitals.[5]

Perspectives for Medical Education

Support for graduate medical education. Graduate medical education has had no financial base of its own; it has grown and proliferated almost exclusively with the support of patient care dollars. In 1984 the Advisory Committee on Social Security recommended that Medicare funds no longer be used to finance graduate medical education. If the federal government were confronted by the potential exhaustion of the Medicare Trust Fund, it might decide, belatedly, to follow this recommendation and use Medicare funds only for patient care.

Most corporations now are attempting to limit their total outlays for health benefits, and this may lead to an attempt to curtail their contribution to graduate medical education. While public and private-sector leaders probably agree that our society must continue to provide graduate medical education with funds adequate to maintain an inflow of well-prepared physicians in the future, the level of support might be considerably reduced. Furthermore, if the view came to be accepted that patient care funds are not the appropriate mechanism for the support of graduate medical education, an alternative would have to be devised. Such an effort might be prolonged and difficult.

It would be irresponsible for government and the corporate sector to repudiate this long-established mechanism for supporting graduate medical education unless and until a satisfactory alternative has been designed and is ready to be implemented. Throughout the economy, the costs of employee training are part of the price that the consumer pays, for the most part unwittingly, except in the case of construction (in the unionized sector), where the subsidy is explicit.

Related to these uncertainties about future funding for graduate medical education are other issues involving sources of capital and research funds, in particular to underwrite the clinical adaptations of new knowledge and new technology. The AHCs, as cutting-edge institutions, have developed many clinical adaptations of prior discoveries in the laboratory for use in patient diagnosis and treatment. The shift to a DRG system of reimbursement surely has exercised a restraining influence on the open-ended purchasing of new technology. The acquisition of technology will be further constrained when the current passthrough of capital costs is replaced by a DRG percentage add-on. Such a shift would handicap AHCs that have recently undertaken or are planning to undertake substantial new construction, such as the major medical centers in New York City. Hospitals that have depreciated most or all of their plant would be in a preferred position under the add-on provision.

These uncertainties about future reimbursement, together with an increasing load of indigent patients, may impede the ability of AHCs to obtain necessary access to capital. In fact, the earlier sales of selected teaching hospitals to for-profit chains were predicated in large part on the belief of their parent universities and medical schools that they would otherwise be unable to obtain the capital they needed to rebuild their obsolescent plants.

Future support of biomedical research. There is no indication that the total amount of federal support for biomedical research will be significantly increased. Moreover, it is increasingly clear that the expectation a few years ago that corporations would become a major new source of funding for biotechnology research at leading research-oriented AHCs was overly optimistic. Some corporate money will continue to be forthcoming, but not on a scale to make a significant difference in the overall level of research funding. A more important source will be the Howard Hughes Medical Institute, whose future grants may approximate $350 million annually over the next ten years.

Income from faculty practice. During the past decade or so, the share of income from faculty practice plans as a proportion of medical school budgets had moved into first place, higher than the contributions of federal or state government; currently, it accounts for just under 40 percent of the total. As a result, an increasing number of institutions report that their swollen clinical faculties are trapped in a situation in which they must devote more of their time to providing patient care to optimize revenue for salaries. Consequently, they have less time for teaching and research.

Scaling down medical education. Consequent to the growing belief that the physician shortage has turned into a surplus, there are certain to be increasing pressures from government, business, and the public to resize the medical education system. If we need fewer physicians, specialists, hospitals, and beds, the existing medical educational structure should be reduced correspondingly to match these new realities.

Governance. New challenges in the arena of governance, broadly defined, in the medical school, university, and medical profession, as well as intersectorially, invite attention and action. University trustees and deans of the medical schools have good reason to look anew at the idiosyncratic position of medical education within the academic community. The first issue that merits close examination is the great disparity in the costs and length of medical education as compared with other professional training, including law, engineering, architecture, and business. Moreover, can a ratio of one professor per undergraduate medical student be justified, or does the ratio conceal the fact that most of the medical faculty are engaged primarily in research and patient care?

Significant reforms in medical education must be closely linked to the reestablishment of a core faculty of relatively small size under the leadership of a dean, with the educational responsibilities of the medical school as their main objective. Trustees of universities that own their principal hospital affiliate would be well-advised to consider removing the hospital to an independent, if closely allied, organization, if only to put more distance between themselves and the hospital, whose continuing financial stability has become increasingly problematic. In short, the university and the medical school should cover the salaries of the core teaching faculty via "hard money." This would go a long way to shift decision-making power with respect to appointments and promotions based on research and practice plan income from department and division heads back to the dean and the core teaching faculty, where it once was vested and currently is vested in all other professional schools.

The other major governance problem relates to the medical school and its principal teaching affiliate. Because of the financial uncertainties that face the future of large teaching hospitals, we noted that it is unwise for universities to continue to "own" their principal affiliate because of the potential risk to the university's endowment. If the teaching hospital is under an independent board of trustees, it will not be easy to appoint a single institutional head to whom both the dean and the hospital administrator are responsible. On rare occasions, the university and the hospital boards may agree on such an individual. Otherwise, the governance of the AHC will require one or more liaison committees competent to address and resolve problems of interest to both parties.

In sum, the substantial elongation of medical education after World War II and the ceding of responsibility for graduate medical education to teaching hospitals, residency review committees, and specialty societies were not the result of considered planning. If medical education is to be shortened, improved, and made less costly—all necessary and desirable objectives—the medical school faculty must be empowered to oversee the educational process from preadmission to first certification.

Recommendations for Reform

Our recommendations generally address three substantive issues: the process of medical education (its structure and duration); the size of the enterprise (number of faculty, students, schools); and compositional elements such as the characteristics of the students admitted and their orientation and expectations. We are aware of the seeming paradoxes in some of these recommendations, most notably our call for a shortened medical education in the face of an ever-expanding knowledge base. All of the recommendations, however, have unity and consistency when viewed in the context of a commitment at all levels of the medical establishment to curriculum changes that reflect alterations in the missions of teaching, research, and financial support of health care delivery. It is not enough to eliminate redundancies in the curriculum or to revise the course load. What is needed is the development of a new curriculum that strengthens the central purpose of medical school training.

Duration of education. At the beginning of this century, medical school graduates were prepared to enter the practice of medicine after one year of internship training at most. Today, they are not. It is now almost universally accepted that medical school graduates need a minimum of three more years of training before qualifying to practice as general physicians. Graduates in law, business, and engineering are considered qualified to practice upon receiving the professional degree. Should not the same be true for physicians? We believe that, with judicious planning, four years of clinical training (rather than the present five), combining the last two years of medical school and the first two years of graduate medical education, are adequate to train a general physician for internal medicine, pediatrics, or family medicine.

One of the advantages of the present system of graduate medical education is the diversity of opportunities available to medical school graduates based on aptitude, accomplishment, and interest. Some of this diversity could be preserved if consortia of medical schools agreed to cooperate in the clinical education of their medical students, particularly during the last two of the proposed four clinical years.

Therefore, we recommend that what are now the last two

years of medical school and the first two years of graduate medical education be combined, and that the medical school assume responsibility for planning an integrated curriculum in consultation with the boards of internal medicine, pediatrics, family medicine, and surgery. We also recommend that this revision in the clinical education of the general physician be implemented by consortia of medical schools rather than individual schools. Further, we recommend that students entering specialties other than general medicine, pediatrics, or family medicine conclude their initial training after three clinical years under the jurisdiction of the medical school. We also recommend that students in the last two years of their clinical training not pay tuition, and receive a stipend similar to present practice in graduate medical education.

Consortia of medical schools. We recognize that any restructuring of medical education involves a variety of constituencies, each with its own special interest. Given the complexities of working through the details of the first recommendation, we believe that one or more pilot efforts would be desirable. Such a fundamental departure from the present structure of graduate medical education should be undertaken by a consortium of medical schools rather than a single school.

Therefore, we recommend that one or more private foundations interested in medical education consider funding several pilot demonstrations designed to test the feasibility of combining the last two years of medical school with the first two years of graduate medical education, with the goal of preparing graduates of such programs for the practice of general internal medicine, general pediatrics, or family medicine. Further, we recommend that prior to launching such pilot demonstrations, a conference of the concerned constituencies be convened by interested foundations for the purpose of advising those participating in the demonstrations on how to finance the final two years of clinical training, including clinical experience in ambulatory settings other than hospital outpatient departments.

Size of faculty. The size of medical school faculties has little to do with the teaching of medical students but reflects instead the personnel needs of the AHC research communities, the magnitude of faculty practice plans, and the size and number of graduate medical education programs. While these are legitimate functions, we think it important to recognize the distinction among them and the fact that not every member of a clinical faculty is simultaneously a fully engaged practicing physician, a dedicated investigator, a committed teacher of medical students, and a conscientious supervisor of residents and fellows. We believe the primary responsibility for organizing the curriculum should be delegated to a relatively small group of faculty members who are paid by the medical school to be primarily teachers and who receive their academic rewards in large part as a result of dedication to teaching medical students.

Therefore, we urge each medical school to reexamine the distribution of effort among members of its faculty and to identify a core group with primary responsibility for the medical school curriculum. The clinical representatives of this core group logically would be drawn, for the most part, from the primary medical specialties.

Flexible admissions policies. Students vary in their interests and in their preparedness to enter into professional education. Some know precisely what they wish to do from the first day of college; others are uncertain after four years of study. Various educational experiments have indicated that early acceptance with delayed admission to medical school can enhance the quality of undergraduate education. Demonstrations also have shown that some students are capable of entering medical school after two or three years of college education.

Therefore, we recommend that medical schools adopt more flexible admissions policies, and that the readiness of the individual be given greater weight than the number of years spent in college. We further suggest that medical schools experiment with early acceptance and delayed admission, to encourage the integration of science education between college and medical school and general education for students who have decided on a medical career but wish to pursue their interests in the social sciences or humanities.

Number of medical schools. Most would agree that today there is a surplus of physicians that is likely to increase. There is simultaneous decline in the applicant pool for medical school and an uneven distribution, so that some schools have far more attractive candidates than they can accept, while others have difficulty recruiting qualified classes.

Therefore, we recommend that each medical school consider

its optimal size in terms of its educational resources and commitment to undergraduate medical education. Further, we recommend that each state legislature that supports in whole or in part one or more public or private medical schools reexamine its commitments to medical education, taking into account the size and quality of the applicant pool, the quality of the educational environment, and how effectively the school or schools are meeting the future physician needs of the state.

More minority students. A significant part of the anticipated surplus of physicians, and particularly the surplus of specialists, has come about as a result of employing FMGs to fill residency positions in teaching hospitals. Since it is in the long-term interest of the public to reduce this surplus of less well-trained physicians, it is reasonable to reduce the number of FMGs who enter the country ostensibly for training but, in fact, with plans to practice medicine here. Given a growing surplus of specialists, it should be possible over time to expand the employment of fully qualified U.S. physician graduates to provide the services now rendered by FMGs.

Therefore, we recommend that residency review committees and specialty boards consider reducing the number of qualified residency positions to approximate the number of American medical school graduates entering the specialties each year.

More emphasis on research. Although the quality of medical education is not necessarily determined by the quality of a school's research program, we are concerned about the decline in the number of physicians interested in research careers, because we are convinced that the physician investigator has certain insights into disease processes that the Ph.D. researcher lacks. From its inception, NIH recognized this, and for a long time underwrote a generous program of training grants.

Therefore, we urge NIH to expand its efforts to interest qualified medical students and young physicians in research. M.D.-Ph.D. programs have been remarkably successful, but there is a need for other pathways for interested medical students or residents if they wish to acquire research experience without having to make a final commitment to a research career. We also urge private foundations interested in medicine to consider seriously the support of research training for medical students and residents as an investment for the future.

Funding issues. The past few years have demonstrated wide

differences of opinion about the future funding of graduate medical education. Recent congressional action that reduced the level of Medicare funding for graduate medical education is likely to be reopened sooner or later. At the same time, there is now virtually no source of funding for training activities carried on at freestanding ambulatory sites, and there is every indication that more and more of the undergraduate and graduate education of future physicians will have to be performed at such sites.

Therefore, we recommend that the federal government, preferably in association with one or more foundations with strong interests in health care, fund a number of policy research studies to explore the ramifications of these educational financing issues with an aim of clarifying the preferred alternatives.

While the reforms that we have recommended involve other constituencies than those directly concerned with medical education, including third-party payers, state and federal governments, the corporate community, and philanthropy, the initiative must come from the leadership of academic medical centers. We hope that the leadership of the AHCs will initiate necessary reforms rather than wait for others to force what might be far less desirable alterations.

The Politics of Physician Supply

The Period of Internal Reform: 1903–1920

A major force that led in 1902 to the reorganization of the AMA, founded half a century earlier in 1847, was the concern of its leadership to raise the standards of medical education. This required the merger or closure of a large number of schools with correspondingly large reductions in the annual number of graduates, many of whom were abysmally prepared to treat patients. What needs to be emphasized is that the AMA took the lead, through the establishment of the Council on Medical Education in 1903, to reduce the number of medical schools and the number of physicians entering the profession. The Council "had been organized primarily to raise the standard of medical education," but its influence was severely restricted until it began to publish its annual evaluations of the individual medical schools including the performance of their graduates on the state licensure examinations.[1]

The AMA's annual evaluation of medical schools began in 1906 and the first report was published the following year. The 160 schools were rated in three categories: Class A (acceptable)—82; Class B (doubtful)—46; Class C (nonacceptable)—32.

As might have been anticipated, these annual published ratings provoked considerable resentment in the medical school community. Accordingly, the AMA in 1908 welcomed the collaboration of the Carnegie Foundation for the Advancement of Teaching in a joint field study of all existing schools under the direction of Abraham Flexner with the assistance of N. P. Cahill, the secretary of the AMA Council on Medical Education.

The report was published in 1910 with Abraham Flexner as sole author. In a lengthy introduction, Henry S. Pritchett, the president of the Foundation, acknowledged the assistance of the AMA and the AAMC, but the Foundation assumed complete responsibility for the findings and interpretations.

Pritchett's introduction calls attention to the two most significant findings of the study:

> (1) For twenty-five years past there has been an enormous over-production of uneducated and ill-trained medical practitioners. This has been in absolute disregard of the public welfare and without any serious thought of the interests of the public. Taking the United States as a whole, physicians are four or five times as numerous in proportion to population as in older countries like Germany.
>
> (2) Over-production of ill-trained men is due in the main to the existence of a very large number of commercial schools, sustained in many cases by advertising methods through which a mass of unprepared youth is drawn out of industrial occupations into the study of medicine.[2]

In his critical Chapter IX, entitled "Reconstruction," Flexner recommended that the 155 medical schools be reduced to 31, a number sufficient in his view to produce 3,500 physicians annually, all that the country would need for a generation or two. Flexner looked to the state licensing boards to bring about the necessary reforms outlined in the report. In his words: "The power to examine is the power to destroy."

The Post-Flexner Era: 1920-1940

Victor Johnson, a later secretary of the Council of Medical Education and Hospitals and a contributor to *The History of the AMA*, assessed the Flexner report, which resulted in a reduction in the number of medical schools from 160 in 1905 to 94 in 1915 and 80 in 1927, as follows:

> These results are encouraging, when it is recalled that the Council had no legal powers, but had to depend upon results through the

establishment of confidence in its findings on the part of government bodies (chiefly the licensing agencies), the better schools, the profession, and the public at large. This confidence was established because of the fairness of the Council's studies, the objectivity and disinterestedness of its approach, and the staunch support of the licensing boards, the Carnegie Foundation and the Association of American Medical Colleges.[3]

In his historical sketch of the Council on Medical Education, Johnson noted that the implementation of the Flexner report created "considerable anxiety . . . lest the diminution in numbers of schools would result in far fewer physicians being graduated and consequently an increasing dearth of physicians in the United States . . . Subsequent events served to provide a certain justification for this fear."[4]

The following table, based on Johnson's data, presents the key figures for selected years:

	Number of Schools	Number of Graduates
1905	160	5,606
1922	81	2,529
1944	77	5,163

In 1925, fifteen years after the completion of the Flexner report, the AAMC organized the Commission on Medical Education "to make a study of the educational principles involved in medical education and licensure, and to make suggestions which would bring them into more satisfactory relationships with the newer conceptions and methods of university education, on the one hand, and with the needs of present-day society, on the other."[5]

The foreword to the final report stated that the work of the Commission was financed by contributions from most of the medical schools in the United States and Canada, the AMA, the Rockefeller Foundation, the Carnegie Corporation, and the Josiah Macy, Jr. Foundation. The Commission consisted of seventeen distinguished leaders of American medicine and education under the chairmanship of A. Lawrence Lowell, president of Harvard University, with Willard C. Rappleye, dean of the College of Physicians and Surgeons of Columbia University serving as the director of study.

The report was published in 1932 at the nadir of the most severe depression in the nation's history, and this may explain the preoccupation with the issue of the surplus of physicians:[6]

> The present oversupply of physicians in this country is likely to lead to unnecessary services, to a lowering of the quality of medical care, and to excessive costs because people are not able to judge their needs in such a highly technical field as medicine.
>
> It is clear that in the immediate past there has been a larger production than necessary and that at the present time we have an oversupply of physicians, although they are not well distributed in relation to the population and to the medical needs of certain areas.
>
> If the United States had the same ratio of physicians to the population as England and Wales, there would be about 82,500 doctors in this country. If the ratio were the same as in Germany the total would be 79,000; France 73,000; Norway 70,000; Sweden 42,500. The actual number at present in the United States is 156,440.
>
> An adequate medical service for the country could probably be provided by about 120,000 active physicians . . . On such an assumption there is an oversupply of at least 25,000 physicians in this country.
>
> There are more physicians in the United States than are needed to provide an adequate medical service for the country. . . . The United States has more physicians per unit of population than any other country of the world . . .
>
> The present medical schools in the United States are producing more physicians than the country needs.

At the same time, a review of the politics of the physician supply in the pre-World War II era, that is roughly from 1900 to 1940, cannot overlook the following discordant notes which continued to be important in the postwar period as well.

· Aggregate figures and analyses of the nation's supply of physicians notwithstanding, many persons living in rural areas, and their political representatives, knew that they had difficulty in obtaining proper medical care because of the inaccessibility of physicians. A communication from the National Grange to the AMA in the late 1920s dealt with this problem.

· There was considerable disquietude among many groups

that raising the standards for medical education made it increasingly difficult for students from low income families to study medicine, an infringement of their right to freedom of occupational choice.

· The reduction in the number of medical schools and admissions placed serious hurdles in the path of various groups subject to discrimination, in particular, Jews and immigrants from Southern and Eastern Europe. Some of the more determined had to pursue their studies abroad.

· The AMA called attention in 1931 to the fact that "the rise of totalitarianism in Europe was beginning to bring a number of physicians to the United States." By the mid-1930s the AMA noted that the number admitted between 1929 and 1934 mounted to 1,916. The number coming from Germany had increased from 22 in 1929 to 160 in 1934. Seven hundred and fifty-five of these physicians had announced their destination as New York.[7]

These references indicate the extent to which the medical establishment—the AMA, the AAMC, the medical schools, deans and key faculty, with strong assistance from interested foundations and the tacit support and approval of the public—were able to determine the flow of students into medicine through the active support of the state licensing authorities.

In a critical study published in 1967, Elton Rayack directed a chapter entitled "The AMA and Medical Education: A Study in Professional Birth Control" to the AMA's policies affecting the physician supply.[8] Though Rayack acknowledged that the 1920s saw a "mildly expansionary" trend in the number of graduates, he emphasized that by 1932 there was a shift to "restrictionism." In 1933 the president of the AMA stated that the country needed only half of the existing medical schools, and the Council on Medical Education urged the AMA to reduce the number of graduates, pointing out that seven schools were planning to reduce their acceptances. Rayack notes that the Federation of Medical Licensing Boards in 1936 suggested a decrease of 500 graduates annually, which in twenty years would reduce the supply of physicians by 10,000. Such a move would clearly contribute to the welfare of future practitioners.

Proof that the AMA was practicing professional birth control is summarized in Rayack's table below:

Year	Medical School Acceptances	Percentage of Applicants
1932–33	7,357	60.0
1939–40	6,211	52.6
1951–52	7,663	38.5

The AMA and its allies clearly succeeded in the 1930s in reducing the number of students admitted to medical school. In the early postwar years the Association continued to argue that not only was there no danger of a shortage, but in fact there remained the possibility of a surplus.

Although the thrust of the AMA's initial efforts to raise the quality of medical education in the early years of this century was not aimed at enhancing the economic position of its members through reductions in the supply of physicians, such a cartel-like objective was clearly manifest in its actions in the 1930s, a posture that carried over into the post-World War II years.

There is no doubt that the virtually blank check given the medical leadership by the public to control its professional affairs led to undesirable policies, in particular, discrimination against applicants to medical school from specific groups held in low social esteem. A recent article by a faculty member of the University of Rochester Medical Center noted that "state medical boards used oral interviews to weed out candidates who were considered undesirable. Some individuals were of the wrong sex. Some were of the wrong race. Others were of the wrong religion. Still others were planning to compete with members of the board or their friends."[9]

One final comment about medical politics in the pre-World War II era. Although the profession deserves credit for its role in raising the standards of medical education, it pursued a highly defensive posture with respect to public policies aimed at broadening access and improving the quality of health care services available to the American public. It invested most of its energies in fighting such changes as expanding health insurance, group practice, capitation plans, and governmental programs that employed salaried physicians to provide services to designated beneficiaries. In the mid 1930s Harvey Cushing, one of the nation's leading surgeons and president-elect of the AMA, wrote to Morris Fishbein, the senior staff executive, advising him to "bury the hatchet about the CCMC (Commission on the Costs of Medical Care) report and take a fresh start . . . to get the profession adjusted to the feasibility of some sort of sickness legislation." Cushing's suggestion was rejected and the AMA maintained its highly defensive posture for the next three decades.

The Impact of World War II

The entrance of the United States into World War II altered many aspects of American life and institutions. Not the least of these were the changes that the war helped to effect in the structure of medical care and in the attitudes and behavior of the American people toward medical care in the postwar era. The following wartime measures were important in terms of their consequences for postwar civilian life.

· The federal government determined the number of young men who were permitted to study medicine during the period of active hostilities and subsidized their education by enlisting them in the reserve forces.

· At the same time the government called to active duty about 40 percent of all physicians in civilian practice. At peak, over 55,000 physicians were in uniform. The fact that the public suffered, at worst, minor inconvenience as the result of this large-scale withdrawal underscored the indeterminate relationship between the number of physicians and the provision of essential health care services to the public.

· Over 15 million soldiers and sailors served during World War II and a large proportion of these servicemen, together with their dependents, were exposed to a higher level of health care services than they had previously known. As a result of this experience their "taste" for medical care was heightened.

· Physicians with specialty certification who enlisted in the War and Navy Departments were commissioned at a higher rank than generalists. This reinforced the drift toward specialization and subspecialty training that exploded at the war's end.

· The management of the expanded army and navy medical departments during the war provided opportunities for many older and younger physicians in uniform to become directly involved in the planning and operation of large medical systems. This experience had a marked influence on their postwar thinking and actions. Three names of such founders suffice: Michael DeBakey, William C. Menninger, Howard Rusk.

· The war years coincided with the dramatic breakthroughs in antibiotic therapies, major advances in surgery, and innovative approaches to the treatment of the mentally ill— all of which set the stage for a heightened appreciation of the potential of modern medicine to enhance the general welfare.

· Millions of Americans relocated to the South and the West as a result of the location of military and naval establishments and aerospace companies in these areas. The decision of many among the relocated population to remain in these regions once peace returned precipitated the need for additional physicians and consequently for new medical schools in such states as California, Texas, and Florida.

· As the war in Europe neared its end in 1944, Congress passed the Servicemen's Readjustment Act (GI Bill), which provided liberal maintenance and educational allowances for those who were discharged honorably from the Armed Services. This set the stage for a large number of returning physicians to undertake further education and training.

· In 1946, shortly after the end of the war, Congress passed the Hospital Survey and Construction Act (Hill-Burton Act), which provided federal assistance to small towns and rural communities to build hospitals in order to raise the level of medical care available to their populations. This was a major departure in federal financing policy, but one that elicited the support of even the conservative leadership in the Congress. It was but one of many efforts that led to the upgrading of the nation's hospital plant and created new demands for additional physician staff. The demand was further increased by the unwillingness of house staff to live in the hospital and serve alternate nights and weekends as had been customary in the prewar years.

· Another important consequence of the nation's wartime experience was the stance adopted by the administration and the Congress favoring the liberal support of biomedical research, which took the form of expanding the National Institutes of Health. In 1940 federal expenditures amounted to $3 million; by 1950 the annual appropriation was around $70 million. The explosive growth of research funding after the war precipitated a much expanded demand for physicians in areas other than patient care.

· A related development, influenced by funding from the NIH (the major source of research support), was the creation and expansion of training programs in various specialties and subspecialties. The directors of these training programs became interested parties in expanding the physician supply.

· The war had demonstrated that many patients suffering from mental illness could be effectively treated. At the war's end major lobbying efforts were undertaken to improve the staffing of state mental hospitals. The NIH eventually made funds available for the retraining of general practitioners, internists, pediatricians, and others who desired to specialize in psychiatry.

· The federal government committed itself at the end of the war to upgrade the large Veterans Administration hospital system in cooperation with the deans and faculties of nearby medical schools. This became a new source of funding for the training of residents and for faculty of academic health centers.

· The war years also provided a major stimulus to the growth of private health insurance (and thereby the growth of demand for medical services) as a consequence of a decision from the War Labor Board permitting trade unions to bargain with employers for health benefits. The Department of Internal Revenue, in turn, ruled that the value of these benefits was tax exempt for employees and tax deductible for employers.

In short, the American people came out of the war with a far more positive view about the potential of modern medicine, with more resources to purchase health care services (via insurance), with the availability of federal funding for hospital construction and research, and with the opportunity for physicians who had served in the armed forces to upgrade their skills by entering or completing residency training supported by GI benefits. The stage was set for a substantial expansion of the health care sector.

In Search of a National Consensus: 1950–1963

President Truman made two unsuccessful efforts during his term of office to get Congress to pass a national health insurance bill. One explanation for his failure attributes it to the strenuous opposition of the AMA and its business allies, particularly the insurance industry; another emphasizes the disinclination of large sectors of the American public to support such a radical departure in the financing and provision of medical services. Although many people at the lower end of the income distribution, in particular those living in outlying areas, had long encountered difficulties in obtaining the health care they needed and wanted, the predominant middle class did not lack access. The principal advocates for national health insurance were a small group of ideologically committed health policy analysts and their followers, most of whom had little political leverage.

Unable to persuade Congress to legislate national health insurance, President Truman asked his Social Security Administrator, Oscar Ewing, to take the initiative to convene a National Health Assembly for the purpose of charting a ten-year program for improving the nation's health. Its report, *The Nation's Health: A Ten-Year Program* (1948), dealt extensively with various deficiencies in the physician supply and the steps needed to overcome them.[10] The highlights of the report with respect to physician supply follow:

> We have only 80 percent as many physicians as we need . . .
> Moreover we do not have enough medical colleges . . .

Our goal for professional health manpower is ... to increase sharply our total professional manpower through training programs and through financial and other support ... increase our present supply of 190,000 active physicians to 227,000 (in 1960) ...

The 12-state yardstick for physicians—the average of the top quarter of the states—is one for every 667 persons. On this basis ... we will need 254,000 physicians by 1960. Our present prospects are for only 212,000 by that date ... the nation will be short 42,000 physicians.

At present our production of physicians is limited by the fact that we have in the U.S. only 70 four-year medical schools with an average enrollment of 335 students each. The average output is about 80 graduates per school for a national total of around 5,600.

At current production rates and taking account of the six new schools being organized we can assume a maximum supply of only 212,000 active physicians by 1960. Increasing our supply to 254,000 actually needed by 1960 would require that we double the training capacity of our medical schools and do this, almost literally, overnight.

The report set a goal of 227,000 physicians for 1960, noted the need to speed the building of six new medical schools beyond the six then under construction, and recommended an initial outlay of $40 million of federal funding in addition to enlarged state and private support.

In the waning years of his administration, President Truman appointed a distinguished national commission headed by Paul B. Magnuson to explore policy alternatives for improving the nation's health care system in the face of Congress's refusal to pass national health insurance. The Magnuson report, issued in five volumes, covered much the same ground as *The Nation's Health* though in greater depth.[11] It recommended emphatically that in order to overcome the financial crisis facing the nation's institutions for educating health personnel, federal funds be made available to modernize and expand existing schools of medicine and make up operating deficits, as well as encourage the development of new schools; to remove the economic barriers which restrict freedom of American youth in gaining entrance to medical education; and to meet the needs for additional Negro physicians.

Despite the strong support of the Magnuson and Ewing reports for federal aid to medical education, the recommendation was blocked primarily by the opposition of the AMA, which feared government encroachment on the education of physicians and the practice of medicine once federal dollars became available to medical schools. A stinging critique of the Ewing report by Frank Dickinson, director of Medical Economic Research of the AMA, provides a succinct summary of the attitudes of the organization toward a broadened role for the federal government in the sphere of medicine.[12]

Dickinson notes that the Ewing report erred in three substantive areas: preventable deaths, the doctor shortage, and the ability of the American people to pay for medical care. With respect to the doctor shortage, he was critical of the assessment on methodological grounds. He argued that the "best twelve-state standard" would inevitably produce a finding of shortage; that the report failed to establish the adequacy or inadequacy of the physician supply in the base year; that it failed to take account of the gains in productivity of physicians resulting from the greater use of auxiliaries; and that it was silent on the question of the relationship between a larger supply of physicians and health status. The critique was trenchant. Nevertheless, Dickinson's identification with the AMA enabled the proponents of an increased supply to disregard his analysis, not only at the end of the 1940s but for the next quarter century.

The AMA was not unaware of the deepening financial difficulties that many medical schools were facing, and the leadership went so far as to signal Congress that it would interpose no objections if the schools applied some of their rapidly growing revenues from recovery of the indirect costs of biomedical research to their educational budgets. The AMA balked only at direct congressional financing for medical education.

In November 1952 Dwight D. Eisenhower won the presidential election with a large majority, and it was clear from his campaign speeches and later pronouncements that he was a true conservative who would aim to reduce the role of the federal government in domestic affairs, moderate the tax burden of the citizenry, and eschew large-scale social initiatives. He was specifically opposed to "socialized medicine," without appreciating the paradox that as a career officer in the Army he had been the beneficiary of such a system throughout his adult life.

It was not until the closing years of Eisenhower's second administration, more specifically following publication in 1958 of the prestigious report of the Secretary's Consultants on Medical Research and Education, that the issue of the scale and financing of medical education again became the focus of public attention.[13] Stanhope Bayne-Jones and his colleagues reported to the Secretary of Health, Education and Welfare, Marion B. Folsom, as follows:

> The Consultants believe that it would not be in the public interest for the number of physicians per 100,000 population to fall below the 1955 ratio of 132 per 100,000. This ratio has remained constant (plus or minus two) over the past 30 years.
>
> To maintain this ratio, the output would have to expand by 1970 to 8700 a year . . . This compares with a production of 6800 in 1956. The domestic output would have to rise by 1900 per year by 1970.
>
> About 1700 additional physicians per year must be produced by new schools . . . Therefore a minimum of 14 and as many as 20 new medical schools will have to be built . . .
>
> Medical schools at this time, and without increasing enrollments . . . require additional operating funds of $10 to $20 million per year. Outside (nonuniversity) support for operating expenses has amounted to millions of dollars per year and not the tens of millions of dollars per year required for optimum performance today and future expansion during the next decade . . .

Since the Consultants included senior executives from DuPont, American Cyanimid, and Eli Lilly, as well as leaders of the medical profession, their analysis and recommendations could not be ignored, even by an administration that sought to avoid new commitments.

Presented with the strong recommendations of the Bayne-Jones report, the Eisenhower administration opted not for action but for another study, which got under way shortly and reported the following year. The Bane report, named after its chairman, Frank Bane, concluded that the mid-1970s would find the country short of between 11,600 and 17,200 physicians and accordingly set forth a series of actions that the federal government should undertake.[14] To quote from its conclusions:

> The maintenance of the present ratio . . . is the minimum essential to protect the health of people in the U.S.

> To achieve this [ratio] the number of physicians . . . must be increased from 7,400 to 11,000 by 1975—an increase of 3,600 graduates.
>
> Expansion of existing, establishment of new schools must be greatly accelerated.
>
> [There is] serious underfinancing of approximately 15 percent of existing schools.
>
> Present schools could add 1,000 [students]; new 2 year schools, 800; 1,000-1,500 at other new 4 year schools. Twenty to 24 new 2- and 4-year schools are needed.
>
> Federal grants in aid [are needed].
>
> More generous public/private support for operating expenses [is needed].

Once again the administration sought to avoid recommending a specific action program to the Congress. And once again, for the third time in three years, it resorted to the establishment of a committee whose report came to be known as the Jones report, taking the name of its chairman, Boisfeuillet Jones.[15]

The Jones report stated unequivocally that the United States faced a growing shortage of physicians and dentists and recommended strongly that the measures outlined in the Bane report be implemented at the earliest possible date. It called attention to a new worrisome factor—the fall-off in the number of applicants to medical school, from 6.6 percent of all college seniors in 1948 to 3.9 percent in 1959, a decline which it attributed primarily to the availability of subsidies for study in fields other than medicine. Withal, President Eisenhower turned over the White House to President-elect John F. Kennedy in January 1961 without forwarding any specific recommendations to the Congress for direct federal support of medical education for the purpose of enlarging the future supply of physicians.

The outgoing administration's stance reflected the unwavering opposition of the AMA to direct funding for medical schools and the absence of any serious support for such an initiative from most professional groups. True, the AAMC had long advocated federal action, but the association was in the process of internal restructuring and was not well positioned to lobby effectively in the final year of the Eisenhower administration. The late 1950s had seen both the Congress and the administration grapple with the costs of acute hospital care for the large number of older citizens and their spouses, people of modest means who, by virtue of retirement from the labor force, were no longer covered by private insurance. Kennedy had campaigned on a platform that favored expanding Social Security to cover the health needs of the elderly population. Early in his administration the president forwarded such a proposal to the Congress where it was tabled in a vote by the Senate. The AMA understood, however, that now that the issue had been placed on the nation's agenda, it would not recede until a solution had been found. For the AMA, resort to social insurance was unacceptable. Accordingly, it regrouped its forces, determined to defeat any new proposal that the administration would present. One consequence of this strategy was the attenuation of the association's opposition to federal support for the construction of new medical schools and student aid so that in 1963 the Congress finally succeeded in enacting the Health Professions Educational Assistance Act, the first program of direct federal assistance to medical schools in the nation's history.

For a decade and a half the issue of expanding the physician supply had emerged periodically on the nation's agenda, only to be withdrawn in the face of unremitting opposition by the AMA, which denied any inadequacy in the present and prospective supply and vehemently opposed direct federal intervention. Nevertheless, during the period of 1946-1963 eleven new medical schools were established, all under public auspices except for the University of Miami and the Albert Einstein College of Medicine of Yeshiva University (New York City). These new schools added 1,485 first-year places to the base year's total, an increase of 25 percent.

The breakthrough that led to federal intervention in 1963 reflected the growing conviction among the public, the leadership of the academic medical community, and the Congress that the shortages in the physician supply represented a present and future danger to the nation's health. It was reinforced by the financial plight of many of the nation's medical schools including such prestigious institutions as Johns Hopkins University. Many medical school deans, with the AAMC as their spokesman, increasingly looked to the federal government as the only escape from financial collapse.

The Federal Government Takes the Lead: 1963-1976

In steering the landmark 1963 legislation through the Congress, Senator Lister Hill impressed upon his colleagues that it was important to pass "basic legislation" immediately and to leave for a later date a large number of related issues. What was first needed was a consensus embedded in legislation that the existing physician shortage was a serious threat to the health and welfare of the American people requiring federal action and the appropriation of sizable new funds. It should be noted that except for long-term funding for agricultural research and veterans, and commitments under the National Defense Education Act of 1958 (in response to Sputnik), the federal government had never been directly involved in the financing of higher education. Thus in 1963 legislation represented a major departure.

With the barrier to federal support of medical education finally eliminated, Congress moved in the years following 1963 to increase the flow of funding to resolve a variety of health care problems that had arisen while the consensus for medical school assistance was gathering.

Two years after the passage of the 1963 legislation, Congress found it was providing money for the construction of ten new schools at the very time that a dozen or so existing schools were nearing the financial brink. Hence in 1965 new legislation was passed including "improvement grants" which assisted the financially distressed schools to stay afloat at the same time that the more affluent medical schools were helped to improve the quality of their offerings.

Brief mention must be made of two other reports. The first was written in 1964 by the President's Commission on Heart Disease, Cancer and Stroke under the chairmanship of Michael DeBakey, and included a special report by a Subcommittee on Manpower.[16] The report stated unequivocally: "The first hard fact is that there is not enough health manpower to meet the needs of the American people. There are not enough doctors and enough supporting people." It noted that the increase in the physician supply barely matched the growth in population. Although it approved in general of the Health Professions Educational Assistance Act of 1963, the report nevertheless pointed out that "it falls far short of the all-out national effort needed to meet a critical national problem—the shortage of physicians." Among the most important of the commission's recommendations was that "legislation be sought to permit forthright support of medical education, this program to include periodic grants to the health professional schools."

The report of the Subcommittee on Manpower included some historical observations:

> The manpower needed for attacking the three great killers—heart disease, cancer and stroke . . . requires expansion of the work force of the entire health establishment. The principal reason for our failure today to maintain the health of millions of people . . . is the paucity of health manpower . . .
>
> We urge that an immediate and massive program be undertaken leading to new construction and enlarged operation of schools of public health, medical and dental schools . . . so that shortages in the health professions will be eliminated . . .

Although the subcommittee supported its recommendations with extended statistical data, it relied primarily on the Bane and Jones reports for evidence that in the absence of special efforts the United States would face a serious shortage of physicians by 1975.

Another landmark report was produced for the AAMC by Lowell T. Coggeshall, a distinguished medical educator, in 1965.[17] Referring to the recently published report of the President's Commission on Heart Disease, Cancer and Stroke, he agreed that "a continuing trend is the growing need for physicians . . . It is clear that more physicians must be trained as quickly as possible and that the result of an increased number of physicians will be 'healthy' not only for the needs of the nation but the profession itself." Coggeshall recommended a reorganization of the AAMC and its assumption of broader and enlarged responsibility, including active advocacy of federal support for medical education.

Three years later, in 1968, Congress acted once again, this time in response to the recommendations of the National Advisory Commission on Health Manpower established by President Johnson in 1966.[18] The commission stressed the importance of broad institutional support in contrast to narrowly targeted categorical grants, in the belief that such funding would provide the deans with greater discretion to determine how best to modernize their curriculum and expand their enrollment. In the amended health manpower legislation of 1968, Congress moved in a number of new directions. Following the commission's recommendation, it enacted a modest "institutional grant" program and also distributed, on a formula basis, additional funds linked to enrollment increases. Moreover, it authorized the Secretary of Health, Education, and Welfare to make special funds available to schools that were confronted with severe financial problems.

Two years later, in 1970, the Carnegie Commission on Higher Education published a special report entitled *Higher Education and the Nation's Health: Policies for Medical and Dental Education*.[19] The report emphasized that "more and better health manpower" was the key to improving the nation's health. It looked forward to the passage of national health insurance within the coming decade, a program which in its opinion would further increase the demand for physicians. Accordingly, the commission concluded, "we see the need for expanding the number of places for training doctors during the next decade by 50 percent."

The commission went on to make a number of suggestions for the restructuring of medical education, noting that the research-oriented Flexner model should no longer determine the medical school curriculum. It advocated strengthening educational efforts in outlying areas and it emphasized the desirability of shortening the years of study required to obtain the medical degree.

The cumulative effects of these six reports and a growing consensus in the administration and Congress that there was a serious physician shortage led to the enactment in 1971 of major amendments to the Health Professions Educational Assistance Act. This legislation introduced the principle of capitation payments to medical schools without making them conditional upon reciprocal additions to the annual pool of graduates. Testifying before Congress, the representative of the AAMC emphasized that in fiscal year 1970, 61 out of the nation's 102 medical schools sought special grants from the NIH to offset financial distress. In 32 instances it was problematic whether, in the absence of such financial aid, these schools would have been able to survive.

Since there was no reliable information about the costs of educating medical students and other health professionals, Congress in its 1971 legislation directed the Institute of Medicine (IOM) of the National Academy of Sciences (NAS) to undertake a comprehensive study of these costs in order to provide a firmer foundation for determining the amount of future capitation payments. The report of the IOM study group, published in 1973, came out strongly in favor of capitation.[20] It argued that medical schools should be treated as a "national resource," since their graduates were mobile and frequently practiced in states other than those where they had received their undergraduate medical education.

From the outset, in 1963, of the federal government's commitment to support medical education, members of the Congress, particularly those from small towns and rural communities, had sought to respond to the growing difficulties that their constituents were encountering in attracting and retaining physicians. Beginning in 1965 with the passage of a student loan forgiveness program, Congress adopted a number of measures aimed at improving the distribution of the physician supply, both geographically and by specialty. In 1970 it established the National Health Service Corps. The following year it initiated the Area Health Education Centers program and also provided special funding for family practice residencies. The first of these efforts provided liberal support for students in return for service in an underserved area upon completion of their training; the second focused on upgrading the skills of physicians and other health care professionals in outlying areas; the third was viewed as a partial corrective to the overspecialization which, in the view of many observers, had come to dominate the education and training of physicians.

In the eight years between 1963 and 1971 Congress had taken a great many initiatives to expand the size and influence the characteristics of the physician supply. A number of actors played key roles in the deepening involvement of the federal government in the support of medical education. The AAMC, spokesman for the medical schools, pressed for direct federal funding for medical education, preferably without conditions. Selected leaders of the medical profession who believed that the output of specialists and subspecialists had gone beyond the point of optimal return advocated increasing the number of primary care physicians, including those to be trained in family practice. The members of the Carnegie Commission on Higher Education lobbied for a large increase in the annual increment to the supply (50 percent). They were joined by voters and their congressional representatives from small towns and rural areas which experienced particular difficulties in attracting and retaining practicing physicians. A substantial number of informed and articulate citizens believed that it was in the national interest to have more members of minority groups study medicine, an objective that could be achieved only if additional federal funding became available for institutional and student support.

The single largest shift on the political horizon was in the position of the AMA with respect to public policy affecting the physician supply. In the April 8, 1968, issue of the *Journal of the American Medical Association (JAMA)*, F. J. L. Blasingame, the executive vice president, authored a special communication on "Physicians and the Market Place," in which he made the following major points:[21]

> The AMA has been subjected to unfair criticism for having limited the number of physicians, whereas the Association has been doing much to stimulate expansion of physician education through helpful legislation, creation of facilities, and a full-scale careers program.
>
> The one thing that has not been done is to put the AMA and public pressure on medical faculties ... to the degree that they will respond to the need. We should be on the side of the public more aggressively in this matter. The benefits of having more physicians are beyond counting ... the quality of care would improve ... the convenience of medical care would improve ... areas that do not now have physicians would be served.

A few years after the reversal in the official position of the AMA on the issue of physician shortage, Boris Senior and Beverly A. Smith argued that the production of more physicians appeared to be an inefficient remedy for the many shortcomings of the existing medical system.[22] More than a decade earlier, in 1960,

I had made the same point in a short note to the *New England Journal of Medicine*;[23] I followed it with a longer article in the same journal in 1966.[24] By that time, however, there were few skeptics left since the AMA was ready to join the expansionists.

During these eight years of growing federal support for medical education, Congress acted on a related front by revising the laws governing immigration into the United States. Although there had been a sizable inflow of foreign trained physicians in the preceding years, the numbers escalated following the reform of the immigration statutes in 1965. By 1972 foreign medical graduates accounted for about 40 percent of all newly licensed physicians.

Although questions were raised from time to time by laymen, physicians, and Congressmen as to the logic and the justification for the affluent United States to be party to a brain drain of foreign physicians, there was no serious opposition to the inflow, in part because many FMGs were willing to practice in locations and settings that could not attract domestically trained physicians. Others provided essential house staff for professionally constrained hospitals. In a period of perceived national shortages, migration from abroad represented a significant increment to the supply of new physicians.

The magnitude of federal support for medical education throughout the 1960s and until 1976 is reflected in the following figures. In 1960–61 the total revenues of U.S. medical schools came to $436 million, of which the federal government contributed $176 million or about 40 percent. In 1975–76 the corresponding figures had risen to $2,389 million and $1,221 respectively; the federal government's share was then 51 percent.

One additional point should be made about the era of increasing federal support for medical education. Despite the dominant role of state governments in the long-term support of medical schools, the federal government's various initiatives were developed and implemented with scarcely a nod in the direction of the states. Washington dealt directly with the medical school establishment. As Michael Millman has demonstrated in his illuminating study, *Politics and the Expanding Physician Supply*, one of the parties of major interest and the largest long-term funder of medical education, state government, was almost totally ignored during these crucial eight years.[25]

Within a few months of the publication of the 1973 IOM report favoring federal capitation on the grounds that medical schools were a national resource, the Assistant Secretary for Health, Charles Edwards, warned the Congress that the nation might soon be facing a physician surplus. For the next two years, 1974–1976, the House and the Senate struggled to find a common base for future federal policy affecting health manpower. They ultimately passed the Health Professions Educational Assistance Act of 1976 which declared the end of the long period of physician shortage. Although it provided for the continuation of various forms of financial assistance to schools and students, the new law took a first step to reduce the inflow of FMGs.

The Emergence of a Surplus

It is not easy to explain the sudden shift from the perception of a continuing physician shortage as late as 1973 to the declaration by the Congress three years later that the shortage was ended. Some of the following factors contributed to the reversal: the increasing output of graduates from new and expanded medical schools; the substantial rise in the number of FMGs; the realization that the new governmental health care financing programs for the elderly and the poor did not expand the demand for services as much as had been anticipated; the disappointment that despite the expansion of the physician supply it remained difficult to meet the requirements of underserved urban and rural areas; and the growing concern with the steeply mounting costs of the health care system.

In 1973 Congress passed legislation providing federal funding for the expansion of HMOs (capitated comprehensive health care plans), in the belief that additional prepaid health care delivery systems would help moderate the steep advances in total medical care expenditures. HMOs cared for their patients with about half as many physicians as fee-for-service practice. Once the expansion of HMOs got under way, as many expected, the demand for physicians would be considerably below the numbers that had previously been estimated.

By the mid 1970s, toward the end of the Ford administration, the federal government had become sufficiently concerned about the explosive growth of the physician supply and its longer-term consequences for the costs and effectiveness of the U.S. health care system that the Secretary of HEW established a committee to review the system of graduate medical education. A year later the new administration of President Carter reorganized this Graduate Medical Education National Advisory Committee, broadened its mandate, enlarged its staff, and provided additional support. The committee pursued in-depth studies utilizing both sophisticated manpower modeling techniques and expert opinion panels. Its report, released in the fall of 1980, concluded that the United States faced a substantial surplus of physicians, over 70,000 by 1990, and roughly double that number by the end of the century.[26]

The Congress and the public received the GMENAC report with indifference, if not neglect, but the medical leadership both in the AMA and in most specialist societies attacked its methodology and many of its findings. Since the administration and the Congress were in broad agreement that the physician shortage had passed into history, they saw opportunities, especially in the face of growing federal budgetary stringency, to reduce substantially, federal support for medical education. The GMENAC report provided support for these budgetary actions. On the other hand, the AMA and the specialist societies were unwilling to accept GMENAC's radical suggestions for significant cutbacks in admissions to medical schools and in the number of candidates accepted into residency training programs.

The critics uncovered soft spots in both GMENAC's methodology and recommendations. They failed, however, to give the report the credit it was due by virtue of the sophistication of its findings, developed by a broad range of outside experts. No quantitative approach to determining the present and future balance between demand and supply with respect to physician personnel could command universal approval. The data could help to point directions for policy but they were no substitute for professional preferences and informed judgments. The medical leadership, however, was not ready in 1980 to come to grips with the complex political issues that the report had placed on the nation's agenda. Given such hesitancy and uncertainty, the leadership opted to attack the report's methodology as its best countermove.

A few specialist societies had earlier been concerned about the size of their residency training programs in the face of a declining workload among experienced physicians; some had taken modest steps to reduce the numbers admitted to training. But no specialist group was willing to move strongly on its own to reduce its future numbers both because of the disruptive effects this would have for teaching hospitals and, more particularly, for fear that in cutting back, they would enable other specialties to gain market position and prestige at their expense.

In the early 1960s the AMA started moving away from its long-held active opposition to direct federal support for medical education. By the late 1960s it had joined the vast majority and favored increasing federal support. In making this about-face the AMA adopted the position that the market could be relied upon to provide the necessary signals. As late as November 1983 the editor of *JAMA* reasserted the principles previously enunciated by the Association's House of Delegates, which provided the framework for the AMA's approach to questions of physician manpower:[27]

> The AMA supports the operation of the self-adjusting market mechanism that is consistent with quality medical care.
> The numbers of physicians should, insofar as possible, be determined by the processes of the market.
> The number of U.S. medical schools should be determined by the availability and allocation of resources and the ability of schools to meet acceptable educational standards.

Earlier that year George D. Lundberg, the editor of *JAMA*, invited me to write a commentary which appeared in the same issue of the *Journal*.[28] My concluding paragraph follows:

> If it is correct, as I believe, that physicians are responsible for about 70 percent to 80 percent of all expenditures for medical care, the AMA must speak out loud and clear in favor of reductions in admissions to medical schools and thereby gain potent allies from outside the medical care system—from government, business, and labor and even the consumer, who is most at risk now that third parties have started to shift more and more costs directly onto him.

Three years later the growing unease of its members forced the AMA to reevaluate its position of reliance on the market to correct the emerging surpluses. At the end of 1986 the House of

Delegates again made a fundamental shift and adopted the position that a physician surplus was imminent and that corrective actions were needed to reduce the number of entrants into medical school and to cut back drastically the inflows of FMGs and USFMGs.

In the six years between the release of the GMENAC report and the newly articulated position of the AMA on the physician supply, modest steps at reducing the inflow of new physicians had been taken by individual medical schools, a few state legislatures, and various federal, state, and voluntary agencies. The reductions, however, proved to be modest. Powerful countervailing forces blocked the redirection of public policy toward reducing the future supply: the need of most medical schools to maintain their tuition revenues, small as they were; the strong local political forces arrayed against state legislatures that contemplated the merger or closure of one or more medical schools; the continuing pressure from underserved communities for more physicians; the recognition that it would be in the nation's interest to encourage more members of minority groups to study medicine; the opposition of white middle-class parents to policies that would make it more difficult for their children to gain acceptance to an American medical school; and the FMG and USFMG lobby and their supporters.

Finally, the preference of the United States to rely on the market rather than on government to shape and reshape the nation's human resources goes far to explain the peripheral role of the federal government in determining the future supply of physicians. But the long era of dominance of the private sector (market and nonmarket forces) may be coming to an end. With annual expenditures for health care in 1989 estimated at around $620 billion, or 11.2 percent of GNP, even a public that prefers the market to government as regulator may begin to have second thoughts, if only because of its interest in decelerating the relentless increase in outlays for health care, outlays that are in no small measure determined by the number of physicians.

The Long View

This eighty-five year retrospective of the ways in which politics have affected decision-making on the nation's physician supply points to the following key actors: the organized medical profession represented by the AMA; the medical educational establishment (AAMC); state government (legislatures and licensing boards); foundations; the federal government; and the voting public. One must quickly add that during much of the long period under review, surely from 1903 to 1940, neither the federal government nor the voting public played any significant role in determining policy directions. The one significant exception was the opposition of state legislators to Flexner's extreme proposal to reduce the number of existing medical schools from over 150 to 31, for fear that so drastic a contraction might leave their constituents without ready access to physicians. But the decision-making power rested primarily in the hands of the medical professionals, who saw merit in implementing most of Flexner's recommendations to reduce the number and thereby improve the quality of U.S. medical schools. The public had no grounds for challenging this cartel-like approach. It too saw advantages to increasing the competence of the physicians who treated them.

The principal sources of friction between the public and the profession in the pre-World War II era related to the difficulties that the rural poor, white and black alike, faced in obtaining physician care. Another was the difficulty that young people from various minority groups faced in gaining admission to medical schools. But neither the poor nor those suffering from discrimination had the political muscle to impact the dominant political forces that were restructuring U.S. medical education during the first half of this century.

The much enlarged potential of therapeutic medicine that marked the post-World War II ear, together with the much enlarged desire of the American people to enjoy the benefits of good health care and their increasing capacity to pay for it, set the stage for a much broader involvement of interest groups in the political decision-making process.

As early as 1948 the Ewing report advocated greater efforts to increase the physician supply and recommended a role for the federal government. Although the Magnuson Commission (1951) supported this policy, the continuing opposition of the AMA joined to the conservative orientation of the Eisenhower Administration succeeded in maintaining the status quo. However, a number of states (and two philanthropic groups) did act during this period to establish new medical schools.

By the early 1960s, with the help of a succession of national commission and committee reports and increasing pressure from a public that was experiencing difficulties in obtaining appointments with physicians, the dam was ready to burst. A key factor was the split in the ranks of medicine. The deans of medical schools wanted and needed federal assistance and many members of the medical profession saw no point in supporting the self-interested behavior of the AMA with respect to federal financing. In 1963 the federal government took its first steps to assist medical schools, and over the next decade its successive actions laid the groundwork for an approximate doubling in the annual output of graduates from U.S. medical schools.

Although the principal thrust of the federal government's efforts was to enlarge capacity in order to assure a much larger number of graduates, it also sought to increase the proportion of students from low income families and from minority groups who were admitted to medical school. Further, the reform of the immigration statutes (1965) made it possible for growing numbers of FMGs to pursue graduate training in the United States and eventually to practice medicine here.

By the early 1970s, surely by the mid-1970s, the long-feared shortage of physicians had given way to a new concern—a prospective surplus of physicians. It took the AMA about a decade to confront the new challenge and to respond. Much the same was true for the AAMC. Neither state legislatures nor the Congress have been eager to step out front and develop policies aimed at downscaling the medical educational plant. The most they have been willing to do is to discontinue support for further expansion.

At a higher level of abstraction, the politics of the physician supply has revealed that the parties of primary interest have been the members of the medical profession and the medical educational fraternity. Further, it has revealed the influence of pseudo-science, inasmuch as most studies of the demand for and supply of physician personnel have proved to be egregiously wrong, often within as short a time as five years.

Finally, one cannot help being impressed by the lack of sophistication of most advocates of an increased physician supply for assuming a direct relationship between the size of the physician pool and the quantity and quality of medical care available to the public. Few perceived the absence of any direct relationship, much less the possibility that more physicians could be dysfunctional.

In sum, history tells a great deal about the changing place of medical care in a market-oriented economy characterized by a long-term resistance to expanding the role of the federal government. It adds little, however, to the formulation of a sensible physician supply policy in a liberal or, more properly, a social welfare democracy.

· 12 ·

Nursing

This chapter will consider what the field of human resources and labor markets can contribute to an understanding of the present nursing crisis, with its shortage of hospital staff and more prospective shortages; explore the changes in the U.S. health care system that have relevance for the future of nursing; and formulate the critical issues with which the nursing leadership needs to concern itself.

The world of work for women has opened up to an extent that is hard for the young to imagine. In 1940 a woman civil servant in Massachusetts, not the most benighted state in the union but also not the most advanced, had to resign from her job when she married. That rule governed all civil servants. The long, severe depression was still blighting our economy, and the unemployment rates were still abnormally high. In the early to mid-1950s, a low point in women's participation in the labor market, two, three, or four out of 100 students at the Graduate School of Business at Columbia were women; today they are 40 percent of the class. When my wife graduated from Cornell, she applied to the Harvard Business School. They wrote back politely: "We are very sorry, but we do not admit women. We suggest that you consider Stanford." The barriers to women's working were high.

The majority of all new entrants into accounting are women. Women account for about 35 percent of all newly licensed physicians: they are not yet 35 percent of the profession, because they have been going to medical schools in large numbers only during the last ten years. In law schools, 40 percent of the students are women. Clearly, a great many career options have recently become available to women; it is the central point about women in the labor market today. Women can now get jobs in practically every sector of the economy and are no longer restricted to only a few fields, such as nursing.

The second point, equally important, is that educational qualifications do not determine salaries in the United States. What they provide is a screen for hiring. The chairman of the Federal Reserve Board, Alan Greenspan, does not have a Ph.D. There are few, if any, conditions for membership in the American Economic Association, other than an ability to pay the dues, which are not high. Wall Street (at least until recently) was attracting top science students from top colleges and universities through high salary offers; it was also attracting a large number of tenured professors. This is another way of saying that education is used as a rough screening device, but that is all it is used for in our labor market. The nurse leadership, however, has stressed more education as the preferred way to raise the status of nursing.

The large corporations have also long been interested in hiring large numbers of young engineers and are willing to pay a premium to assess their potential. Within five to ten years a relatively few move up into managerial positions or into advanced technical assignments, but many others fall back into quasi-technician jobs—proof again that more education may not be the answer to enhanced professional status. For many occupations such upward-and-downward mobility is typical.

A profession coincides with an occupation in only a few cases: medicine is the preeminent one. Among lawyers, for example, many never start to practice law. Others may practice for a few years but then wander off either into business or into a governmental position. This is the American model. Europe is different. The key question in the United States is not what kind of degree you have, but what kind of a salary you earn. In Europe, a person's work, salary, status are heavily determined by prior educational achievements.

Employers are constantly trying to improve their production processes by altering the combination of labor, and within the labor elements, trying to substitute less costly for more costly labor in order to reduce their total costs. As managers, that is also what hospital directors are hired to do: not to make nurses happy, not even to improve the nursing service, but to make sure that patients who come into the hospital are treated effectively and at the lowest possible cost to the institution. Improving the environment for hospital nurses may ease the present and prospective shortages, but administrators must also be concerned about costs.

The U.S. economy is increasingly a service economy, but good service is the exception rather than the rule. Yet three out of every four jobs are in the service sector. In the early 1900s, when he was president of Princeton University, Woodrow Wilson invited a young professor to join. But, he wrote, "I am sorry that I cannot offer you a large salary. I can offer you $3,500 a year, but this will enable you to keep two in help." Two in help on $3,500 a year! Most Americans today, even some wealthy ones, do not have even one in help. Personal service is a thing of the past; institutional service is often unsatisfactory. Good service is rare and very expensive. The notion that more and better nurses could provide better nursing is sound. The question, however, is, who will pay for better nursing?

Every occupational group or profession frequently faces a simple dilemma. On the one hand, to improve the economic circumstances of its members, it is sensible to control its numbers. The medical profession, surely through the 1930s and even later, followed such a policy. On the other hand, an inherent obligation of a responsible profession is to respond to the public's need for services, and that frequently means increasing the supply of practitioners. Yet the biggest barrier to improving the economic returns of its members is for a group to press for increases in the supply. The nursing profession has never faced this problem in these terms.

Two groups are useful for comparison with nurses: teachers and engineers. In the 1950s the country had a severe teacher shortage, the consequence of many adverse conditions, including low pay. Teaching was not an attractive occupation, not even for those who enjoyed their early years in the classroom. If they did not want to go into administration, they could not advance. This is a prototype of the nurses' story. But the Ford Foundation, with the support of various teacher organizations, decided that the answer to the teacher shortage was to increase the supply, thereby insuring that the wage levels would not respond nearly as quickly or as strongly. In the case of the engineers, the corporations which hire large numbers of them had no doubt as to how to proceed. They kept pressing the engineering schools to increase their output because they wanted to have access to a larger supply at a lower price. They were absolutely clear on this. A small group of "consulting engineers" understood this game and opposed admitting more students to engineering schools. The case of nurses is more complicated because there are several routes into the profession. The question of how many nurses we need is not easy to answer. But there is something contradictory in a policy that both advocates expanding the supply and insists on raising the salaries and benefits and improving the long-term career prospects for all nurses.

The U.S. labor market, unlike most other economies, is characterized by high mobility. People move back and forth from academic work to government work to corporations; generals even become presidents of universities. All kinds of movements go on in the U.S. economy. Thus even though about half of all engineers are out of technical work at the end of fifteen years, they do not disappear from the profession. Although they are no longer engaged in technical engineering, they become salesmen or consultants. The United States is also uniquely permissive in terms of its immigration policy, the legislation of the eighties notwithstanding. One of these days the area which extends roughly from Houston to San Jose is likely to become no-man's-land between the United States and Mexico. In any case, we are again resorting to immigration to bring additional nurses into this country. But the recruitment of nurses from abroad is not an aberration. The National Academy of Sciences is deeply concerned that more than 50 percent of all doctoral candidates in engineering programs in the United States in 1987 were foreigners!

Those who succeed in getting better salaries, more benefits, better career opportunities, are those who possess labor market power. That means that a profession or an employed group is in a position to extract above average returns. In times past, automobile workers received good wages from General Motors and Ford because these firms were making a lot of money. They paid their workers well to avoid strikes and kept them reasonably content. The medical profession has been able to earn high salaries because its members alone are permitted to practice medicine. The only way a group gets differentially higher returns is through exercising power in the labor market, directly or through their employers.

The *New York Times* noted that North Shore Hospital, located in an affluent area of Long Island, which has had a long-term relationship with New York Hospital, offered newly graduated RNs up to $30,150 as an opening salary in 1987. The applicant must have a bachelor's degree and accept shift work. The experienced (2 years) RNs were being offered $34,150 plus additional compensation for clinical specialization. Now, North Shore is a rich community in Long Island, and that is what its hospital can offer. In the same newspaper the Veterans Administration Hospital in the Bronx offered nurses $28,000 as the opening salary. Both are located in the same metropolitan area. Clearly the depth of employers' pockets is an important factor in determining nurses' salaries.

Earlier mention was made of the relatively short working life of many teachers and engineers. In nursing the conventional statistics, based on those who maintain their licenses, suggest a high retention rate for nurses. But it would make more sense to include in the base all nurses who graduated, including several hundred thousand who no longer bother to renew their licenses because they do not contemplate going back into nursing. Moreover, no other "profession" has as many part-timers as nursing. Lapsed licenses, temporarily out of nursing, and part-time employment do not speak to a high order of professionalism.

Admittedly many fields have employees with short work lives. Consider the armed services: a young man enlists for one or two terms, eight years or so and then he's out. After twenty years of government service one can retire, often on a good pension. Mention was made earlier of engineers with a work life of fifteen years. When it comes to nursing, one must distinguish different age cohorts. Nurses in the future will not necessarily replicate the patterns of labor force attachment that have characterized nurses who entered the profession in the 1960s and even less those who entered in the 1950s.

Finally, it is important to realize that in many fields, in fact in most, higher earners are concentrated in administrative and managerial positions: those who remain in operational assignments are left behind. There is little likelihood that a nurse who remains in bedside nursing for twenty years will be able to earn as much as a nurse who has moved into administration, unless she were to become a clinical specialist with broad responsibilities.

The health care system, like the labor market, sets bounds on nursing because its major payers, the employers and the government, are under pressure to contain costs. Another limit on nursing is that the hospital industry is a mature industry, and we probably have at least 150,000–250,000 excess beds in the system. Sooner or later, if we finally succeed in doing something about cost containment, a considerable number of hospitals are going to close. They will probably be mostly small ones, although New York City closed quite a few good-sized hospitals in the 1960s and 1970s.

Although skepticism is called for concerning all efforts aimed at reforming our health care system, we are seeing a big push toward managed care, with HMOs, PPOs, gatekeepers, and the federal government trying to capitate Medicare patients. There is reason to question whether any or all of these efforts will transform our current system. But it is reasonably certain that the reforms under way will prevent individual billing by health professional groups, including nursing, whose members cannot bill at present. We are moving in the opposite direction. Explorations are under way to establish fee schedules for physicians. Clearly, a major push is on to reduce the scope of individual billing, not to extend it.

Both Congress and HCFA agree that the initial base for DRGs was set too high and the best way to recoup for overpayments is to have HCFA severely constrain upward adjustments in the reimbursement rates for Medicare patients. Less, not more, money will be flowing into the system. At the same time there has been an explosive growth in new administrative and control mechanisms affecting admissions, payment, quality of care, and so forth, which has created a new demand for nurses to fill these administrative slots. Since most of these new jobs involve records of one sort or another, nurses who understand medical terminology are the preferred employees for these openings. Here is another form of competition to bedside nursing. We are probably some way from the peak of this new demand.

Another fact that affects nurses is that the supply of physicians continues to increase. Consequently, their salaries are lower and the competition is stiffer. Physicians are feeling the stress of a health care environment that seeks to maximize health care and minimize costs. When a group begins to lose its power, it becomes defensive. It is not therefore likely that physicians as a group will cooperate in improving the status of nurses.

The nursing leadership thus needs to ask itself hard questions. What evidence is there, for example, that this new shortage of nurses is significantly different from earlier ones? Increasing numbers of women have been entering the labor market for several decades. It is true that the demographic profile is somewhat less favorable for young, white women coming of working age. But a caveat is needed. Every day that the economy continues to expand brings us one day closer to a recession. No one knows how long the recession will last or how deep it will be. How much of a recession do we need before the current shortage recedes even if it doesn't evaporate? The present economy is not chiseled in stone and contains no guarantee that the current expansion will continue much longer.

But even if nursing is experiencing a new kind of shortage, what are the key dimensions worth worrying about? It is reasonably certain that North Shore Hospital will have all the nurses it needs, even if it has to pay each one $40,000 per year to fill its ranks. It may have trouble in attracting a specialist nurse for night duty or on a holiday weekend, but that is probably the extent of the trouble that this particular hospital will face.

The United States is a big, diversified nation, and conditions differ not only among regions and states, but often in districts within the same city. One needs to specify where the critical shortages are or are likely to develop. When hospitals and physicians find that patients need care and there are not enough nurses to provide it, they will resort to alternative ways of providing the required care. To talk about the nursing shortage in general is not illuminating. True, we could use several hundred thousand additional nurses in our nursing homes. Many, probably most, elderly institutionalized persons are not receiving the level of care that they need. But the taxpayers will not pay for it, so there is little point in talking about this facet of the shortage problem. As long as we have no intention of paying for adequate numbers of nurses for nursing homes for the poor elderly, there is no effective demand for them. One must specify more carefully just what is meant by a critical shortage. The conventional answer is: a critical shortage means budgeted funds are available to cover the costs of hiring additional nurses, but they cannot be found.

Nursing has remained primarily a white profession. Black nurses are less than 7 percent of the total. The proportion of blacks in the American economy is closer to 11 percent, and the population of blacks among the young people coming into the labor market is closer to 13 percent, which means that nursing has about half its appropriate representation. If the shortage is real, which is the underlying postulate, one must work to redress racial imbalance. Admittedly ghetto schools don't prepare youngsters properly for high school graduation or for admission to community colleges, but if the nursing shortage is truly acute, it is necessary to build bridge programs that offer interested young people in the black community—and older persons as well—an opportunity to enter a nursing program.

A career in nursing offers good prospects for young people from socially constrained environments. An opening salary for a graduate of a two-year community college is in the $27,000 range and may shortly rise to $30,000, which is attractive in terms of competing salaries. Many more young people from low-income backgrounds are or will be interested in studying for a nursing degree. They may not represent the best and the brightest, but they are capable of earning an AA degree and performing effectively as bedside nurses.

The nurse leadership has been unhappy that the nurse practice acts have not been radically expanded, but attacking that issue is not likely to pay off. Nursing lost out when the nation moved to produce many more physicians. The nursing leadership at the time was too timid to stake out a larger place in the health care system. Now, when there is a surplus of physicians, an effort to broaden nurse practice acts will be fought by the medical profession every inch of the way. Unfortunately, it will be difficult for the nursing profession to find allies at a time like this, when government and business are interested in one facet of health care, and one facet only, and that is to control the amount of new money that they must put into the system.

Despite the strong advocacy of the nursing leadership, there is little prospect that nursing education and licensure will be differentiated between those with a baccalaureate degree and the nurse technicians with two years of college education. The major stream of new entrants into nursing are graduates of two-year programs, and there is little or no prospect of a change in this pattern, especially in an era when admissions to baccalaureate programs are dropping and a number of four-year nursing schools are closing. Moreover, the nursing leadership has never explained satisfactorily, particularly to those who run hospitals, the advantage of having nurses with baccalaureate degrees assigned to bedside nursing. The administrators of the almost 6,000 acute care hospitals are willing to pay less than a dollar an hour extra for two years of additional education. Clearly nursing needs a reasonable number of well-educated nurses, but not necessarily for assignments to bedside nursing.

A suggestive question is whether nursing has anything to learn from engineering education, which is specialized at the college level. One graduates as a mechanical engineer, an electrical engineer, a civil engineer, and the graduate seeks a position that matches his specialty training. If a shortage of clinical nurse specialists develops, it might make sense for nursing at the baccalaureate level to take a hard look at the multiple tracks of engineering education.

It is clear that night and weekend shifts for nurses and the lifestyles of the American public simply don't jibe. As a consequence nursing must rely on a large number of part-time workers. But since many hospitals are being transformed into intensive care units, they need nurses—or some alternative caregivers—around the clock to care for their seriously ill patients. The more education a nurse gets, before or after she begins to work, the quicker she leaves patient-care duties. Nursing has been stressing fringe benefits in the form of subsidized education, but these benefits accelerate the flow of nurses away from bedside nursing. This dilemma is not restricted to nursing. In the Army, many field grade officers who have had an opportunity to acquire higher degrees often take early retirement and find civilian jobs. This is the logic embedded in broadening peoples' choices. Better educated persons try to take advantage of new career opportunities.

The nursing leadership confronts increasingly difficult situations in providing adequate care for seriously ill patients. It needs to look beyond the single perspective of nursing to explore alternative ways of delivering the needed services with fewer, not more, baccalaureate-trained nurses. This leads to two further questions: who will decide, in the face of worsening shortages, how best to cover patients' nursing needs? Will it be the hospital administrator or the senior nurse or both, working together with the physician staff? And how much money will the American public put into improving the salaries and status of nurses in the face of the nursing crisis?

In view of the foregoing analysis, the nursing leadership must review critically what worked and what did not work during the years when nursing had many things going in its favor. Because nursing was not able to solve its occupational and professional problems when the environment was favorable, it faces a more exposed and difficult situation today. In the early 1960s it would have been relatively easy to expand the number of nurse practitioners. At that time physicians would have helped or at least not stood in the way. They were making so much money that nurses were no threat to them. But the nurse leadership failed to move. They were unable to unify their ranks.

The leadership needs to assess how the labor market and the health care systems have been changing, to project how they are likely to continue to change, and focus on the implications of these changes for nursing strategies. The fight for more power, more money, or more autonomy for nurses will not get easier; it will get tougher. The real earnings of workers since 1973 have failed to increase: the only reason that families are somewhat better off is that most of them now have a second member in the labor force. And we have been borrowing huge sums from abroad. For nursing to get a big slice of new money in such a constrained environment will prove very difficult if not impossible.

Wages for nurses are going up; they always do in the face of shortages, but nursing will find it very difficult to achieve large-scale transformational changes. The American people may be friendly towards nursing but the tough question is whether they will back that friendliness with more cash and other good deeds.

· IV ·

Patients' Needs
and Resources

Clinical Decision-Making
in Catastrophic Situations

The elderly are by no means the only sector of the population to face catastrophic situations, although their plight is perhaps better recognized and publicized. Under the medical care system in the United States, support for the elderly who have acute care needs is quite different from the support for those who require extended nursing home or home care. Even so, the support for the elderly is much broader and deeper than that for children and adults whose medical condition does not qualify them for inclusion under Medicare. In view of the unbalanced federal budget, it would not be feasible to introduce new legislation aimed at bringing about equality of access to health care to all patients facing catastrophic costs for their treatment. Instead, private sector efforts to provide insurance for the elderly who require long-term nursing home or home care should be aggressively pursued.

With money lagging need, it seems desirable, given the affluence of many of the elderly, to tie new benefits (such as catastrophic coverage) more closely to the individual's ability to pay. Congress has taken steps in taxing half of the Social Security benefits of those beneficiaries who have a tax liability, and recently adding to the tax liability of those elderly on Medicare who pay income tax; a similar approach ought to be followed with respect to Medicare, particularly Part B, where the proportion of beneficiary payments (27 percent) is far below the original congressional intent of 50 percent.

Another aspect of the treatment-money confrontation touches on the issue of whether the individual physician should be forced to deal with questions involving the costs of alternative treatments. The allocation of scarce resources is a macro-problem to be decided at the societal or institutional level; it should not be added to the tasks incumbent upon the individual practitioner. He or she has to do the best for his patient. To be sure, rationing of scarce resources is, and has always been, a part of the U.S. health care system. But it is necessary to distinguish between the rationing that occurs as a result of inequalities of private income and public resources, and explicit systemwide rationing aimed at controlling the total outlay of health care dollars. It is possible, even probable, that high-tech medicine will continue to be the driving force of the health care system, and therefore the time may come when explicit rationing can no longer be avoided. In that event, the criterion of "anticipated life expectancy" is better than age as the basis for determining who should have the opportunity to live. However, in the case of patients eighty-five or ninety and above, age alone might be a reasonable criterion for making certain close-call decisions about the use of scarce resources.

Money plays a key role also in choices affecting neonates whose life prospects look questionable or bleak. Since society currently makes only limited assistance available to parents who confront the task of raising severely handicapped children, extra weight ought to be given to the decision of parents who request their physician not to take Herculean steps to save the life of their defective baby. It seems inherently unfair to saddle parents with the lifelong care of a hopelessly defective child in the face of society's unwillingness to make a reasonable contribution to such an onerous responsibility.

On the whole, governmental interventions should be avoided in critical decision-making regarding efforts to prolong life or the termination of life supports. It is far preferable to leave the decision to the individual, to surrogate decision-makers, the attending physician, and the hospital's rule-setting body. One exception to the principle of nonintervention by government would be on a point where medical practice has reached broad agreement, such as the definition of brain death. In such a case there might be an advantage to giving it the added support that comes with governmental laws or administrative regulations.

In a democracy such as ours, where citizens hold widely conflicting values about life and death, it is incumbent upon the medical profession and others in a position to influence medical decision-making (hospital administrators and trustees, and so forth) to be sensitive to such conflicts and not to act in high-handed disregard of the sensitivities of those with an opposing view (the Baby Doe case). The recently established Biomedical Ethics Board could serve as a forum for the analysis and assessment of complex medical-ethical issues. Such a forum and others at state, local, and institutional levels could, over time, go far to reduce the conflicts that stem from differing value positions. Important professional bodies, such as the American Medical Association and the American Bar Association (together with other national organizations), could likewise work together on some of the problems in the medical-ethical arena and, where possible, perhaps arrive at a national standard.

Is the "cost of dying" also a public policy issue? Experts such as Ann Scitovsky claim that the cost of dying has not been a significant, and certainly not an overriding factor in the acceleration of medical care costs. It is true that people incur relatively high costs in their last year of life, particularly in the last six months of life. But no data support the widely held belief that the dying are subject to very high cost interventions. In fact, the opposite appears to be true. Most of the elderly who die receive less intensive treatment than younger patients who die. However, it is easier for a terminal patient to escape high cost interventions if he can be cared for at home or in a hospice rather than in an acute care teaching hospital, where the style of practice is to do more, not less. On the other hand, a dysfunctional aspect of the current DRG system is the incentive to hospitals to discharge dying patients even though they can not be properly cared for at home, only to readmit many within a short time.

The political power of the elderly, as expressed by strong lobbying efforts and large turnouts at the polls, has been a major factor in accounting for the substantial gains they have achieved over the last quarter-century. In contrast, no comparably well organized bodies exist to advocate for greater and better efforts to meet the health and other needs of disadvantaged children. In a democracy such as ours, which tends to respond to pressure group tactics, the uneven constellations of those advocating on behalf of the elderly and those advocating on behalf of the young can result in gross imbalances in policy and programs that persist over long periods of time.

Many problems of catastrophic proportions are connected with the rapid growth of the AIDS population. Most of the victims are in the age group of twenty to forty-four, and aside from Medicaid and public hospitals, there is no support system currently in place to respond to their needs for a substantial amount of care—not only acute care, but also nursing home, home, and chronic care. With their medical costs from diagnosis to death likely to be in the $50,000 to $75,000 range—and with the certainty that more and more people will be stricken with AIDS—the absence of a financial support system only adds immeasurably to their difficulties and to the difficulties that the American people will face as we seek to respond to the needs of these victims. If any further evidence of the deficiency of our current social insurance system for medical care is wanted, one need only add AIDS patients to the neonates.

Despite the foregoing shortcomings that include, in addition to AIDS patients and neonates, individuals who incur catastrophic medical expenses for nursing home and home care, more public expenditures for medical care was not necessarily the best answer to the unmet health needs of the American people. More outlays for education, housing, even food might result in greater societal benefits.

Areas for research that may improve decision-making in catastrophic situations are as follows:

· Learning more about the subsequent quality of life of neonates who have been the "beneficiaries" of elaborate medical interventions.

· Using whatever acceptable "preventive" devices exist that hold any reasonable promise of reducing the number of individuals who would otherwise be exposed to the AIDS virus.

· Learning more about the efficacy of such instruments as the "living will" in guiding medical decision-making at the point when the seriously ill elderly are faced with treatment alternatives.

· Clarifying the cost-benefit of high-tech interventions to elderly sick individuals and to society.

· Making an extensive study of the potential and limitations of treating seriously ill patients in their homes which would assess not only direct financial costs but total social costs, including loss of earning capacity for the family caregiver.

· Planning studies that would calculate the costs of broadening Medicare to provide "catastrophic illness coverage" to persons under 65 including the rapidly growing AIDS population.

· 14 ·

Rationing Cancer Care

The conventional wisdom in the United States is that health care is not rationed. But all economies—communist, socialist, welfare, and capitalist—must ration. They differ only in the instruments which they employ to accomplish their objective of allocating scarce resources among competing needs. A capitalist society such as ours, relies heavily on "the market" to perform the rationing, is restrained from doing so in the case of health services because of the prevailing social ethic that holds that all individuals, irrespective of their ability to pay, must have access to essential care. Hence approximately 70 percent of all health care expenditure is provided by government and insurance, which contribute roughly 40 percent and 30 percent respectively.

Providing access to essential health care for the entire population is no mean task in a country of 240 million people distributed over 50 states which differ widely in their economic wealth and in their political attitudes to the role of the individual versus communal responsibility. The quality of health care available to different groups in the population, and particularly to the poor, varies greatly between the urban population of the Northeast (New York) and the rural population in the South (Mississippi and Alabama). Much of the difference can be traced back to availability of resources and government financing, but differences in medical practice, social mores (racism), and philanthropy—to mention only three factors—must also be taken into account.

The dynamic nature of the health care system implies that

there will be no ready consensus about what constitutes "essential care." The more rapid the additions to knowledge and the rate of technological innovation, the greater the variability in medical practice. In part, it reflects access to resources such as the latest imaging devices or knowledge of and access to the newest chemotherapeutic agent, but is also a function of the age, training, and experience of the specialist directing treatment.

Essential Care for Patients with Cancer

One way of looking at the costs of caring for cancer patients and placing these costs in context is to compute the overall expenditures for cancer, which amounted in 1980 to just under $11 billion or about 2.3 percent of the total outlay for the nation's health care.[1] About two-thirds of the outlay for cancer care went for hospital treatment, 23 percent for physician services, 5 percent for drugs, 4 percent for nursing home care, and 1 percent for other professional services. These data suggest that any significant reductions in the costs of caring for people, once they have been diagnosed as having cancer, are directly linked to reductions in hospital admissions and surgical interventions.

Evidence of the relatively narrow margin available for significant reduction in the cost of caring for cancer patients is found in data from the Surveillance, Epidemiology and End Results (SEER) program of the National Cancer Institute (NCI). SEER findings for the period 1973–1982 indicate that 62 percent of all admissions for cancer undergo surgery, and for 43 percent, surgery is their first and only treatment; the remaining 19 percent receive radiation, chemotherapy, and hormone therapy singly or in various combinations as adjuncts to surgery. Thus a reduction of any consequence in total expenditures of over $25 billion for the care of cancer patients could be achieved only if the number hospitalized and operated on were to be substantially reduced. Three distinct but related propositions must be considered: are too many cancer patients being admitted to hospitals; are too many operations being performed on cancer patients; are there less costly sites where cancer patients can be treated effectively?

Surgery remains the treatment selected for most cancer patients whose tumors have not metastasized. While oncologists may differ as to the preferred treatment plan for any particular patient (a decision which in any case requires the agreement of the patient), surgeons who practise in sophisticated health care systems have no plans to reduce operative procedures for cancer. Moreover, since Medicare (1966) there has been a pronounced increase in the number of patients over the age of sixty-five who have been admitted to hospitals for evaluation, treatment, or care when they are in a terminal stage of cancer.

Since the introduction by the federal government in 1983 of prospective reimbursement for hospital care based on DRGs, hospitals have been under increasing pressure to admit only those patients for whom in-patient treatment is essential, and to discharge them as soon as they can be safely moved to a less intensive setting such as a nursing home, hospice, or their own home. Investigation had suggested that alternative care in a hospice setting would, on average, be less costly than care in an acute hospital with intermittent care at home or in a nursing home. As a result, Congress acted in 1982 to provide hospice care as a Medicare-reimbursable benefit. Cancer patients who are judged to have entered the terminal stage of their disease (defined as a six months' life expectancy) may seek admission to a hospice as an alternative to further treatment in an acute hospital.

It should be noted that the United States has seen a considerable growth in the number of hospice beds over the last years in different settings—independent facilities, set-aside beds in general hospitals, or other types. These beds are under nonprofit or for-profit auspices and (unlike some British counterparts) do not depend primarily on volunteer workers. With regard to the nursing homes as alternative sites for the treatment of the seriously ill and the terminal cancer patients, good nursing home care in most areas in the United States is severely limited, and the cost approximates $100 a day or more. Some nursing homes which provide a minimum of services have fee schedules in the $35 per day range, but would resist accepting terminal patients who require frequent medication and considerable nursing care. Nursing homes, therefore, provide only a limited back-up support system for the treatment of severely ill and moribund cancer patients.

Many cancer patients, even those who are terminal, continue

to live at home, with the acute care hospital serving as the back-up. But the care of the terminally ill patient at home generally imposes heavy burdens on the caretakers—occupational (conflict with work), financial, emotional, and physical. Moreover, while home care systems are being expanded and improved, for the most part they provide only limited amounts of skilled nursing and other types of professional care. In addition, most physicians prefer not to make house calls.

The acute care hospital thus remains the primary resource for treating patients who require diagnostic evaluation and surgical or nonsurgical interventions (such as initiating drug regimens). However, current hospital reimbursement policy is seeking to reduce the inappropriate use of the acute care hospital for those who are not in need of intensive care. Alternative sites—hospice and nursing home—are providing more care than previously; nevertheless, most cancer patients continue to live at home and receive medical care on an ambulatory basis from their physician or the out-patient department of a nearby hospital.

The Auditing of Patient Care

During the last two or three decades Congress has taken several steps aimed at encouraging the medical profession to improve its auditing function. The stimulus for such action came from the belief that PSROs would exercise peer pressure to influence the practices of physicians who were making excessive use of hospital facilities by admitting patients who did not actually require inpatient care, or by retaining hospitalized patients for excessively long periods. More recently, Congress and the HCFA, which administers Medicare, have emphasized the need for the successor PROs to give attention not only to the use of resources but also to the quality of care the patient has received.

The performance of common surgical and medical procedures often varies in frequency three- or fourfold among neighboring communities with similar epidemiological profiles. It is therefore not surprising that it is difficult to achieve a consensus as to the most effective ways of treating cancer—a disease where diagnosis is often complicated, treatment protocols variable, and the outcome under any of the accepted treatment modes uncertain.

The popular press in the United States periodically reports on cancer patients (usually those in advanced stages of the disease) who travel to foreign countries to undergo some new or unorthodox treatment regimen. These determined patients argue that since they have nothing to lose, they should not be deterred from turning to new and still unproved therapies, which they want available in this country. Similar attitudes apply in resorting to drugs that are prescribed abroad but have not been licensed by the FDA for use in the United States. Again, a small but significant number of cancer patients seek admission to major Clinical Cancer Centers in order to be accepted into an experimental treatment program. These trends suggest that in an open society in which no single authority is in a position to determine treatment protocols, auditing the treatment of cancer presents considerable problems.

The American courts are moving rapidly to enlarge the scope of decision-making for the individual to determine the types of medical treatment that he is free to accept or reject, including the prerogative of refusing treatment which might prolong his life. Since cancer therapy often entails complex trade-offs involving length of life, quality of life, disfigurement, and so on, and since individuals differ in their risk/benefit preferences, standardized treatment protocols are not possible.

Screening

There is broad agreement that the earlier a cancer is identified, the greater the prospects in most instances that the appropriate intervention will prolong life, even if it cannot cure the cancer. One would infer that increasing resources should be directed to screening populations at risk in order to increase longevity, but there are a number of problems attached to screening that may or may not be compensated for by assumed gains resulting from the extended years of life.

Screening that involves all or substantial sectors of the population on a regular basis will lead to substantial increases in current outlays. There are also the risks that may attach to the screening procedure, such as increased exposure to radiation at mammography; perforation at sigmoidoscopy; erroneous positives and negatives; failure to allow for the regression of lesions (cervix and breast); and the difficulty of using averages to convey the value of screening to a particular individual.

The results of D. M. Eddy's meticulous cost-effectiveness studies strongly support screening of breast, colon, and cervix,[2] and the American Cancer Society[3] provides cogent evidence for the following types of screening:

- Colorectal tests: digital rectal examination every year after age 40; stool blood test every year after age 50; and proctosigmoidoscopic examination every 3–5 years after age 50 following two annual examinations with negative results.

- Pap Test: annually until two successive negative tests, then once every 3 years.

- Breast cancer detection: monthly self-examination by women 20 years and older; physical examination every 3 years from ages 20 to 40 and then every year; baseline mammogram between ages of 35 and 39, every 1–2 years between 40 and 49, and every year for asymptomatic women age 50 and over.

For patients who see their physician at least once a year, some of the foregoing tests carry only modestly increased outlays but others, such as sigmoidoscopy and mammography, often carry price tags of between $100 and $200. In the mid-1980s about 32 million women were above the age of fifty, and disregarding the relatively small number who currently follow the ACS recommendation of an annual mammographic examination, the screening costs for this one procedure for this cohort would be approximately $3 billion each year. A review on screening for breast cancer[4] concluded: "Nationwide screening for breast cancer is desirable, although at the present time we have insufficient data to select entrance ages, periodicity, and utilization of risk factors." This does not appear to be the strongest basis for an incremental investment of $3 billion!

Surveys have shown that a considerable number of individuals, particularly those with a low income, have no regular source of medical care and rely on the emergency room or the out-patient department of a neighborhood hospital or a community clinic. Members of this "unconnected" population, probably of the order of one out of every five individuals, are likely to encounter a different physician, often a resident in training, every time they seek medical attention. The lack of familiarity of the examining physician with the patient, and the patient's limited ability to pay for care, make any form of screening not directly connected with presenting symptoms highly improbable.

Prepaid medical plans, a rapidly growing form of health care delivery in the United States, have long emphasized their concern with prevention, but it is difficult to assess how extensive their screening procedures are. An important consideration is that their enrollment so far has consisted primarily of members of the work force and their dependents. Under the stimulus of Medicare some prepaid plans have recently been enrolling numbers of the post-65 population. If this enrollment shift in favor of the elderly is sustained, it remains to be seen whether prepayment plans will intensify their screening programs for cancer and other major diseases.

Health Education and Prevention

There are a number of actions that the public can take to reduce its risk of developing cancer, and the American Cancer Society has listed eight measures of primary prevention. As one would expect, avoidance of cigarette smoking heads the list because it is so heavily implicated in lung cancer, accounting for about 30 percent of all cancer deaths. Nutrition comes next, with warnings against obesity, high fat diet, consumption of smoked foods, and heavy use of alcohol, while emphasis is placed on the beneficial properties of high-fiber foods, foods rich in vitamins A and C, and cruciferous vegetables. Too much exposure to sunlight, to the use of smokeless tobacco, to estrogen replacement therapy, to diagnostic radiation, are also singled out as dangers to be avoided. The final category comes under the heading of occupational hazards, and includes such industrial agents as nickel, chromate, asbestos, vinyl chloride, and so forth.

Although some targets of primary prevention such as smoking fall within the scope of the individual's decision-making, others, such as exposure to industrial agents, usually do not. In some cases the exposure is not unequivocally bad: for example, the use of radiation or estrogens to achieve important health gains are instances where gains need to be weighed against potential dangers. The law and administrative action may be essential in order to reduce exposure to occupational hazards or they may be helpful in discouraging the use of cigarettes through taxation or in the designation of nonsmoking areas.

It must be noted that once people become dependent upon cigarettes and alcohol or acquire certain food habits, the costs of modifying their behavior are far greater than if they had not become addicted in the first place. As evidence of progress, one can observe that the campaign against smoking has had considerable success in the United States and has resulted in a decline of over 20 percent in the case of men, and over 12 percent in the case of women, during the last decade. X-ray technology has been significantly improved, physicians are more cautious with respect to the prescription of estrogen therapy for menopausal women, and the federal and state governments are trying to improve control of occupational and environmental hazards.

The list of known or potential carcinogens is very long and each year it lengthens, yet great differences of opinion continue to exist as to the amount and intensity of exposure that will place the individual at risk of contracting cancer at some point in his life. There are also great difficulties in assessing the multiplicity of risks in an industry that makes extensive use of potential carcinogenic agents. And the costs of forcing an enterprise to cease operating or forcing a community to relocate are so great that they cannot be advocated unless the evidence is overwhelming.

Research and Private Sector Initiatives

It is not easy to determine how much money is enough when it comes to investment in research, particularly investment in basic research, which is the principal focus of the NIH. The total NIH budget in 1985 was in excess of $5.1 billion, of which the NCI received about $1.2 billion, but over the decade of the mid-seventies to mid-eighties the proportion of the proposals approved by its peer review committees that the NIH has been able to fund has been decreasing. The ratio of awards to approvals had declined from its former level of two out of three to a low of one out of three. It is worth noting that in addition to funding by the NIH, cancer researchers received about $70 million for their projects from the American Cancer Society (ACS) and that directly and indirectly, their work is also assisted by sizable philanthropic grants.

Since the late 1960s there has been rapid growth of for-profit enterprise in the delivery of hospital and health care (the production and distribution of pharmaceuticals, medical supplies, and appliances have always been concentrated in the private sector). The private sector now has a growing role in the financing of biomedical research, particularly in response to the new opportunities in biotechnology. In 1985 the research expenditures of industry were approximately equal to that of the NIH, each contributing just under $5 billion of the total of almost $13 billion. Other divisions of the federal government accounted for an additional $2 billion and the remaining $1 billion represented state and local outlays, and philanthropic efforts.

It is important to review these initiatives of the for-profit sector and its much stepped-up investment in new biologicals that might prove effective in the treatment of cancer. Acknowledging that new immunological agents are now "state-of-the-art treatments," Stuart E. Lind[5] raised some worrying questions: Who will look out for the patient? Will access to information about these treatments be restricted? Are conflicts of interest inherent in this type of work? Will patients' access to medical treatments be restricted by the ability of companies to patent? How do we resolve the issue of equal access to care? Is it fair to ask the patient to be a partner in the research enterprise? When, if ever, is it reasonable to ask patients to pay for the development of treatment-related research for their own immediate benefit?

Conclusion

By the end of the 1980s total health care spending will have increased from the $425 billion level of 1985 to $620 billion or more. Although many groups have been vehemently advocating "cost containment" since the early 1970s, the result has been largely talk. The only retrenchment that can be observed is cutbacks in access to health care for the poor and the uninsured, although fortunately these have not been profound.

No serious consideration has been given to the rationing of cancer care, nor is there likely to be, given the positive orientation of the American public to science and technology. The major issue in 1987 was the level and direction of federal support for cancer research, and many saw the growing involvement of the private sector in applied research as a favorable development to compensate for the decreased rate of growth in federal financing.

A few issues related to rationing stayed on the policy agenda: How aggressive should physicians be in the treatment of so-called "hopeless patients"; should terminal cancer patients be cared for in sites other than acute care hospitals; does it really make sense to have all women over fifty undergo mammography every year; what criteria should govern public policy in reducing carcinogens in the workplace and the environment? But these questions aside, the United States in 1987 was not seriously considering the rationing of cancer care.

· 15 ·

Health Care for the Elderly

This chapter examines the many complexities involved in thinking about health care for the elderly, on the ground that conceptual weakness will inevitably result in poor policy. True, sound policy also requires a commitment to humane values, but in the absence of sound conceptualization and analysis any policy will flounder.

To begin with, the concept of "health care" itself needs to be clarified. A homebound person receives assistance three times a week for several hours from a home health aide who does the shopping and helps the disabled person take a bath. Is this health care? Or: many persons are maintained in nursing homes that do not employ registered nurses around the clock or schedule regular physician visits for assessment of the changing health status of the residents. Is this health care?

Nor is the concept of "the elderly" perfectly obvious. Is it an arbitrary designation that covers all persons above the age of 65, or should it be reserved for a narrower band, say the group 75 years and older or even 85 and over? For example, in some respects, including their pattern of utilization of health care services, the "young-old," persons between ages 65 and 74, more closely resemble persons between 55 and 64 than the "old-old," persons over 85.

Considerable uncertainty and disagreement characterize the selection of chronological age criteria for dealing with the elderly. The Social Security legislation was amended several years ago to raise the age of entitlement to full benefits from 65 to 67; several states have moved to eliminate age as a factor in terminating employment; and it is increasingly common for surgeons to operate on patients who have passed their eighty-fifth, even their ninetieth, birthday.

In the absence of chronological criteria it is difficult, often impossible, to establish objective criteria for societal and organizational decisions, such as the time that the chief of surgery of a teaching hospital should be asked to step down, or the time that an individual should become eligible for his or her pension. Furthermore, reliance on any "objective" criteria leaves much to be desired. In an effort to reduce personnel, more and more American corporations have resorted to an early retirement strategy that encourages executives to leave at age 55, and sometimes even earlier. Social Security provides for retirement benefits to begin anywhere from the age of 62 to age 70, with payments adjusted to age.

How do we take account of variations in vitality and performance among members of the same age group, as well as between the young-old and old-old? A significant minority of the old-old keep working or are otherwise engaged in purposeful activities until they die, and they remain substantially free of disease and disability, suffering no loss of function other than a reduction in physical vigor. At the opposite extreme are individuals whose health has so deteriorated that they are housebound or bedridden and require constant care. These contrasting conditions are found among the old-old, and to a lesser degree also among the young-old.

It is therefore important to avoid gross generalizations about the health status of the elderly. Although aging is associated with an increase in chronic illness and other disabilities, most people are able to continue the activities of daily life independently or with modest support from others. Even among the old-old, only a minority are in nursing homes, and some are substantially free of impairment.

Furthermore, during the last two decades, the elderly in the United States have made marked gains in income and access to health-care services, as a consequence both of federal programs and of increases in personal financial assets. Significant improvements in federal programs include substantial increases in benefits received from Social Security, the indexing of these benefits to compensate for inflation, the introduction of Supplemental

Security Income for the needy elderly, the growing proportion of persons retiring at age 62 or 65 who are entitled to partial or full benefits, and special provisions for those below the age of 62 who are permanently disabled. Further improvement in the economic position of the elderly has resulted from increases in private pensions, home ownership, and savings.

In terms of cash income alone, the proportion of persons 65 and over who fell below the poverty level declined from over 35 percent in 1959 to 12.6 percent in 1985.[1] In recent years, the federal government has also introduced and enlarged transfers in kind—medical and nursing care, food, housing, and related benefits. When these are taken into account, the proportion of the elderly below the poverty line in 1985 dropped, according to the lowest of several estimates, to 3.2 percent. Only one in thirty of all elderly persons was living in poverty.[2]

As other chapters of this book make clear, the period since the early 1960s has seen real improvements in the income, health services, and social supports that have been made available to the elderly both by federal and state governments and by private pension plans and enhanced personal savings. The absolute and relative improvements in the position of the elderly have outpaced those of any other demographic group, notwithstanding the continued shortfalls in income, health care, and social services for particular subgroups.

Unresolved Problems

The generally improved economic position of the elderly must not obscure severe deficiencies in various dimensions of their lives. A small minority continue to live in poverty, even after receiving various services in kind. A much larger number escape the definition of poverty but have incomes less than twice the poverty ceiling. Half of all the elderly are found within this income range. The most vulnerable group are women living alone: about 2 million, or more than one in four, live in poverty. Among the aged who live alone, five times as many women as men subsist below the poverty level. These unattached women account for more than half of all the elderly living in poverty.[3]

Furthermore, despite the broad entitlement and coverage provided by Medicare, a small number of the aged, those who encounter catastrophic illness, remain financially vulnerable. This explains the amendments adding catastrophic insurance to Medicare.

By all accounts, the two most serious shortcomings in the present structure of health care financing for the elderly relate to nursing home services and home health care. Skilled nursing home care costs in excess of $100 per day. Medicare has very restrictive conditions governing eligibility and reimbursement for such care; Medicaid pays only for those who are without financial means. As a result, elderly persons who do not qualify for Medicaid because their income and assets exceed the ceiling must pay for their care themselves or look to their children to cover their nursing home costs. Obviously, only the wealthy and those on the upper end of the income scale can afford an annual bill of $25,000 or more for nursing home care that they may need for several years.

Many of the elderly can remain in their own homes, provided they have assistance in the performance of daily activities, such as shopping, cleaning, and bathing. Here, too, the Medicare program is very restrictive, providing services only to persons who require concomitant nursing or other professional care for a defined medical condition. Again, persons who are not eligible for Medicaid must cover such outlays themselves or seek financial assistance from their children. Annual expenditures of $5,000 to $10,000 for part-time assistance and of $25,000 for full-time care represent a financial burden that only a small minority of families can meet, especially when help is required not for a few weeks or months but for several years.

In summary, a small minority of the elderly lack even the minimum income that would make their last years bearable, and a great many more—about half of all those over 65—subsist close to the margin of poverty. This means that they can live reasonably well as long as they are not confronted with a basic change in their circumstances, such as the need for assistance in the performance of their daily activities or admission to a nursing home.

Professionalism and Consumer Choice

In the United States, the individual states long ago devolved onto the medical profession a high degree of responsibility. Self-regulation, in turn, enabled physicians to play key roles in determining how health care services, both in-hospital and ambulatory, were delivered to the public. For example, President Lyndon B. Johnson concluded that it was the better part of political wisdom to reach an agreement with the AMA specifying that Medicare would not alter the traditional physician-patient relationship. Accordingly, the federal government agreed to reimburse physicians for the care of the elderly on a fee-for-service basis, with rates determined by the UCR standard—usual, customary, and reasonable.

For Medicaid, the states were not required to follow federal policy on physician reimbursement, and many of them soon placed a low ceiling on the amount that they would pay for an office visit. As a result, a substantial proportion of physicians, especially those in large cities, overtly or covertly refused to accept Medicaid patients, or at most were willing to treat only a selected few. This forced many of the indigent to seek care from the emergency rooms of neighboring hospitals or from "shared practices" (Medicaid mills), usually staffed by physicians with the least training and competence.

The practice of home visits by physicians was largely discontinued with the onset of World War II. Although Medicare Part B will pay for house calls, until recently most of the elderly have found it very difficult to be treated at home. The rationale offered by physicians has been that adequate medical assessment cannot be made without the use of the sophisticated, nonportable equipment found in their offices or in the hospital. The marked increases in hospitalization of the elderly in the post-Medicare period reflect this style of practice, and the trend is reinforced by the ability of physicians to see more patients and bill at a higher rate when services are performed in the hospital.

On any one day, almost double the number of patients are found in nursing homes (roughly 1.4 million persons) than in acute care hospitals (750,000).[4] Nevertheless, except in the best of the long-term care facilities, physicians are conspicuous by their absence. Many of the residents do not undergo a medical examination from one month to the next, sometimes from one year to the next, and without proper diagnosis and treatment, many deteriorate unnecessarily.

Medical school training in the United States concentrates on diagnosis and treatment of the acutely ill, with little emphasis being given to care of the chronically ill. Professional bias among care providers and the absence of suitable reimbursement for nursing home visits thus go far to explain the low level of medical care received by many of the institutionalized elderly.

Furthermore, since for a long time Medicare paid hospitals on a cost-reimbursement basis (which even for a few years included a 2 percent override to help finance innovations), hospitals became the principal beneficiaries of the much enlarged flow of federal funds. As more elderly patients were admitted and their treatment was intensified, federally covered hospital expenditures increased rapidly.

Nursing homes, most of them under private ownership and management, attracted a large part of the funding made available through the Medicaid program. As owners opened new homes or expanded existing ones, beds were rapidly filled by elderly persons, who themselves sought to be admitted or whose families urged their admission in order to be relieved of the continuing burden of their care.

Decision-makers concerned with Medicare and Medicaid have always been reluctant to approve a broad program of reimbursement for home health care on the grounds that, once they start down this road, the substantial contributions made by the patient, members of his or her family, and neighbors would be withdrawn in whole or in part, and large additional costs would be shifted to the public purse. In recent years Medicare has increased its reimbursements for home health care services, but it has kept tight controls over such payments so that they continue to represent only a small percentage of total Medicare outlays.

Organizations that lobby for the elderly have been pressing for reforms in the structure and financing of health care services that would permit the deployment of public funds to help aged individuals remain in their own homes rather than be forced to enter nursing homes. However, despite growing interest in and out of Congress, only minor adjustments have been made to expand Medicare. Advocates for the elderly have understandably been unwilling, except in the case of hospice care, to "trade" a lower level of reimbursement for acute care in favor of alternatives to such care. Congress is concerned that, without such trade-offs, broadening entitlements for nonhospital care will be additive, not substitutive, and, in the face of large future deficits, it is unwilling to take the risk. Congressional caution has been reinforced by recent reports from the General Accounting Office (GAO) that found no clear-cut evidence of net savings from the experimental programs it reviewed. The GAO suggests there may even be the risk of higher total costs from an expansion of alternatives to hospital care.[5]

The critical issue is that no societal mechanism currently exists to rationalize the flow of expenditures for health services for the elderly among the complementary settings of home, nursing home, hospice, and acute care hospital and to provide the optimal amount of care for the available dollars, giving due consideration to the preference of the elderly for remaining in their own homes as long as is feasible. The search for a rationalizing mechanism has been inhibited by the strong resistance, overt and covert, of influential providers and funders such as federal and state governments, acute care hospitals, nursing homes, and physicians, to serious experimentation that could threaten their entrenched interests.

Organization, Financing, and Resource Use

Unfortunately, the difficulty of altering the present flow of resources for the provision of health and related services to the elderly goes beyond the resistance of interested parties. To begin with, health care must be delivered to people where they reside. This means that the federal government can never ensure that all beneficiaries will obtain the services to which they are entitled under the law, because it cannot ensure that a physician will be available to treat them, much less that he will not overcharge them.

Although the federal government pays between 50 percent and 78 percent of all Medicaid costs, state governments regulate such critical matters as the capacity of nursing homes, methods of copayment by families, and the fee schedules of physicians. In recent years, in order to reduce expenditures, the Department of Health and Human Services has authorized waivers giving state governments greater latitude to control expenditures while maintaining or improving the quantity and quality of care. In areas of the country where local government plays an active role as funder, gatekeeper, and provider of services to the citizens who are dependent on public dollars, responsibility is divided between the state and local bureaucracies.

These organizational complexities extend beyond the interrelations among the several levels of government. The great majority of nursing homes are under private ownership and management: of the almost 26,000 nursing homes in the United States over 21,000 are privately owned.[6] Even allowing for the fact that the remaining facilities under public and nonprofit auspices have, on the average, larger capacity, the private sector controls over two-thirds of all nursing home beds.

The tensions arising out of the division of responsibility among those who finance, provide, and control health care services for the elderly are reflected in the recent actions of many state governments to limit the expansion of nursing home beds through the use of certificates of need. State governments have discovered that available nursing home beds invariably become filled. Hence one way to limit the state's costs for nursing home care is to control bed capacity.

Another source of tension between state governments and private providers of nursing home care has been the reluctance of most states to make use of their licensing authority to control effectively the quality of care that is provided. Aside from the costs of inspection, which are high when homes are inspected annually, many states have hesitated to decertify and close nursing homes that fall below acceptable standards, especially in areas with long waiting lists. Politicians believe that the citizenry generally prefers a lower level of care to a total absence of care.

Complexities also arise in dovetailing the responsibilities of the individual patient and his or her family with the government's responsibilities for the financing of care. The issue is directly joined in the case of patients who can remain in their own homes on the condition that they receive assistance in performing their daily activities. Medicare will reimburse for such personal care services only if they are required in conjunction with a recognized therapeutic service, such as nursing care or physical therapy. As a further example of these complexities, recent revisions in the Medicaid regulations of several states, including Massachusetts, Maryland, and New York, mandate a larger contribution by the family to the costs of nursing home care for individuals who require it.

Most governments have been unwilling to broaden eligibility under Medicaid to include personal care services because they recognize that such care is currently paid for by the patient or members of the patient's family or is voluntarily provided by family and friends. Municipal government in New York City is the outstanding exception. With support from the state, it has put together funds from a number of sources (including Medicaid) to provide home health care for 40,000 persons, at a cost of approximately $800 million annually. In Britain, greater flexibility in commingling public and private funds for the care of the homebound elderly permits local authorities to pay for relief workers or for the short-term transfer of patients into residential facilities to provide a respite for family members.

Equity and Ethics

Under contributory pension systems, many individuals who die prematurely or soon after they retire receive less from the system than they have paid in. Others who live well into their seventies or longer receive much more in benefits than they have contributed. This situation has not led to conflict in most countries because the younger generation recognizes that if government did not cover the minimum needs of their parents, the residual responsibility would fall on them. They realize further that sooner or later they too will be among the elderly and will have to depend on the system for some part of their support. Potential conflict has been further attenuated because economic productivity has risen, and the total pool of goods and services available for distribution has increased during most of this century. The elderly, who have contributed to enlarging the stock of human and physical capital, the basis of productivity gains, have an indisputable right to share in the enlarged income available for current consumption.

However, conflicts have arisen and will arise in the future about the appropriate share of national expenditures that should be allocated to meet the income and health care needs of the elderly. The long bout with inflation and the recent retardation in the rate of economic growth have contributed to these conflicts. A continuing problem has been the fiscal integrity of the public pension systems. In many European countries, legislatures are aware of growing strains in the financing of pensions. Nevertheless, politicians, loath to unleash the wrath of the elderly, have preferred to delay taking corrective actions. In the United States, Congress amended Social Security to reduce current and prospective benefits only in 1983. It remains to be seen whether these changes will provide the long-term financial solution that has been claimed for them.

The American social welfare system was structured with a major concern for equity. The initial Social Security legislation was intentionally skewed in favor of the elderly, who would be most in need of government assistance to maintain even a minimal standard of living. In the succeeding decades, many amendments to the system have been particularly sensitive to the needs of those who leave the labor force without adequate retirement income. As noted earlier, major progress has been made to ensure that through entitlements and means-tested transfers, all of the elderly will be able to live above the poverty level.

However, favorable evaluation of Social Security in the United States and of most public pension systems abroad should not obscure the tensions that exist between entitlements and means-tested transfers. Many persons who have supported themselves throughout their adult lives are loath to seek "charity" in their later years. For example, a significant proportion of the British elderly do not claim the supplementary grants to which they are entitled, and many people in the United States who could qualify for Medicaid or other means-tested benefits do not apply for them.

Since almost all public pension systems include a wage-related component in the determination of benefit levels, those who have held low-level jobs and have an intermittent employment record—notably women—are likely, once they retire, to receive an amount that is insufficient to maintain them at a reasonable standard of living. There does not appear to be any way of ensuring that all persons receive an adequate pension without means testing. If the economies of the developed countries experience a period of sustained growth, it may be possible in the future for all persons to receive an adequate pension at retirement. In the interim, however, means testing cannot be avoided.

Many developed countries have long operated a national system of medical insurance that provides access to hospital treatment for all persons, the elderly as well as those of working age. However, law or custom often limits the amount and quality of medical care provided for the elderly. In the United Kingdom, where hospital financing has been most constrained, the elderly have been subject to two types of rationing. Those who do not require emergency treatment must join a queue and wait their turn for elective procedures. Since many of the elderly suffer from chronic rather than acute conditions, they account for a high proportion of those in the queue. Furthermore, in the United Kingdom, as in many other European countries, expensive new interventions such as open-heart surgery, renal dialysis, and hip and knee replacements are not uniformly available to the elderly on the grounds that these costly procedures should be limited to persons in the younger age groups who are likely to benefit the most from them.

Once a society explicitly restricts the total amount of its resources allocated to therapeutic medicine, it is difficult to fault a rationing policy that favors the younger age group, but this does not put the matter to rest. Does a civilized society with a reasonable command of resources have the right to deny the elderly life-extending and pain-reducing treatment while still spending large sums on defense, recreation, or cultural activities?

An acceptable policy is difficult to formulate and to carry out, even when the society, such as the United States, has made a commitment to furnish the full panoply of modern medicine to all persons, including the elderly. Yet how sensible is it to engage in heroic interventions to keep alive patients, including the elderly, who are unlikely to regain a significant degree of function or the ability to care for themselves? Those who favor the present practice of maximal care for all argue that one can decide only retrospectively, not prospectively, whether medical intervention is justified. But the issue remains acute because approximately 25 percent to 30 percent of all Medicare expenditures are incurred by patients who die within twelve months.[7]

The formulation of standards and procedures for determining whether and when to institute or discontinue life-prolonging interventions for the elderly and other patients who are moribund represents a major challenge. The growth of "right to die" movements reflects the concern of many citizens that they, or their legally responsible relatives, be consulted.

Pressures on the System

Skeptics who argue that recent revisions of Social Security will not ensure its long-term financial stability may prove to be right, if the American economy becomes plagued once again by a combination of rapid inflation, slow economic growth, and a sustained high level of unemployment. Even barring this unfavorable constellation, the Trust Fund may not have the necessary resources to meet its obligations to the large number of beneficiaries who will become eligible after the year 2010, when the baby-boom generation begins to reach retirement age. The prospective rise in the retirement age to 67 will help to moderate the financial pressures on the system so long as there is no increase in longevity, which would work to offset these gains. However, unless the world economy—of which the United States remains the leader—should collapse, unfavorable economic conditions are not likely to undermine the Social Security system within the remaining years of this century.

The outlook with respect to health care for the elderly, however, is less propitious. The Reagan administration early on signaled the Congress that programs for the elderly need major changes in policy and financing, and its record during its years in office has shown some successes and some failures. In seeking to moderate federal outlays for Medicare patients, the administration's major success was the establishment of prospective reimbursement for inpatient hospital care, which has been associated with substantial declines in hospital utilization (although it was not the cause of these declines). However, it is too soon to predict whether the new DRG system will in fact enable government to control effectively its outlays for medical care. The most recent projections of the HCFA give no basis for optimism.

The Reagan administration also moved to encourage HMOs to enroll Medicare patients and made modest changes in payment systems for physicians' services, graduate medical education, and capital costs. However, its proposals to substantially increase copayments by Medicare beneficiaries were defeated, and it was unable to win congressional approval to place a ceiling on the federal contribution to Medicaid.

During these same years, many states took the initiative to cut back their Medicaid programs, but the plight of many of the poor and near-poor in obtaining essential health care services and the more buoyant economy since 1983 have led to a reversal of this policy; in fact, many state governments have actually expanded the number of Medicaid-eligibles. However, states continue to limit the expansion of nursing home capacity, with the result that many of the sick and frail elderly experience increasing delays in gaining admission.

As of late 1987, the overall picture relating to health care for the elderly was neither rosy nor gloomy. No new money materialized to underpin a large-scale expansion of nursing home capacity or a significant improvement in the quality of nursing home care. Furthermore, no significant new money came in to broaden Medicare (or for that matter Medicaid) entitlements to effect a major increase in home health care. Both programs are likely to expand, but only with private, not governmental, dollars. There may conceivably be some new governmental funds available for nursing home and home health care if current expenditures for hospitalization of Medicare beneficiaries can be redirected. However, this is at best a promise.

Directions for Future Health Care Policy

Total expenditures for health care for the elderly amounted to almost $120 billion in 1984. The major categories of expenditure, in descending order of importance, hospital care, nursing home care, and physician services accounted for approximately 85 percent of the total. The remainder went for dental services, other professional services, drugs, and insurance. Thus, for a population of almost 27 million persons age 65 or over, the per capita expenditure amounted to $4,200, which is about equal to the average sum that each retired person received from Social Security.[8] The critical questions are, what can be done to improve the prospects for more and better services for the sick and feeble elderly, and what actions would worsen the problems that they face?

On the positive side, it is important for the elderly to maintain the broad access to acute care hospitals so that they will be able to receive the benefits of therapeutic medicine. There may be opportunities, however, to avoid heroic interventions, not only to reduce dollar outlays but also to contribute to the ease and dignity with which the individual confronts death. In this vein, the recent expansion of hospice care warrants continuing evaluation to determine its potential for easing the difficulties that patients and their families experience when recovery is no longer possible.

Although the demonstrations of community-based care for the elderly have not yet yielded positive results—at least not in terms of total dollar savings—they must be continued in the anticipation that cost-effective models will emerge that will enable more of the frail elderly to continue to live at home. On a related front, research into the causes and the treatment of incontinence and senility among the elderly should be intensified. These two conditions contribute greatly to the demand for nursing home care.

As of the end of 1987 private insurance companies, sometimes with state assistance, were beginning to look more seriously at writing insurance for long-term care. It will probably require considerable experimentation before reliable results emerge and it may turn out that private companies will never write policies for individuals and families of modest incomes and assets. But the result should not be prejudged.

For a long time there was much discussion but little action on permitting Medicare beneficiaries to convert their entitlement into vouchers that would enable them to enroll in an HMO and thus secure comprehensive health care coverage. The federal government moved slowly and few HMOs were interested in opening enrollments to the elderly until they could get a better idea of the unknown risks. Although each of the parties has become somewhat more venturesome, it will take several years before evidence accumulates about the interest of beneficiaries in joining and the willingness of HMOs to accept them. What is clear is that the federal government is willing to move ahead and reimburse HMOs at 95 percent of average adjusted costs for Medicare beneficiaries. What remains unclear is whether the government will benefit. It could suffer financially from adverse selection if the healthier elderly should opt disproportionately for HMOs, thereby increasing total Medicare expenditures.[9]

Recent efforts by the financial community to develop new ways whereby the elderly may turn their ownership of a home into an income stream for use during their last years can turn out to be an important factor in narrowing the gap between income and need. About 70 percent of all Americans own their homes, and most of the elderly no longer carry a mortgage. Hence they can look forward to a significant increase in their annual income through a reverse annuity mortgage.

The continuation of present inpatient hospital benefits, together with greater opportunity for the elderly to join HMOs or to be treated in hospices in the event that they become terminally ill, seem, at least for the near term, to be assured. On the other hand, there will be at most only modest government initiatives to enlarge nursing home capacity and home health care other than through "savings" realized by cutting back on the current scale of inpatient care. Such savings will be hard to achieve.

The standoff between additional governmental resources and the unmet, growing needs of the elderly brings us face to face with the central theme formulated at the outset of this chapter: the necessity of combining new knowledge with humane societal values in the task of selecting among competing policy goals and alternative methods of implementation. The mid-eighties have witnessed moves in many different arenas—federal, state, and local—directed toward reducing the gap between the needs of the elderly for more and better health-care services and the inability or unwillingness of most governmental units to increase their appropriations for this purpose.

President Reagan's successful effort in 1981 to reduce federal expenditures for domestic programs, coupled with his willingness to permit the states greater discretion in determining the specifics of their Medicaid programs, led many states to reassess their nursing home programs and to slow down the growth of nursing homes. This measure of economy coincided with growing opposition from many groups of elderly persons to be shunted into nursing homes as the only means of receiving support services. The elderly much prefer to remain in their own homes and communities. It is essential, therefore, to continue the experimental programs that are now in progress to assess the feasibility and the costs of maintaining more of the sick and frail elderly in noninstitutional settings.

Under the best of circumstances some of the sick elderly will need institutional care, and therefore the states must ensure adequate capacity. Two radical proposals also merit attention and study. First, the federal government, in association with a representative group of states, should explore whether any significant gains can be achieved by prospective merging of Social Security, Medicaid, and other governmental programs as a means of enlarging the resources available for expanded institutional care.

Second, and even more important because of its scale and potential, private carriers, employer groups, and nonprofit organizations, such as the AARP and foundations, should explore programs and mechanisms whereby middle-class families and individuals might be able to insure themselves for extended nursing home and home health care.

The last years of the Reagan administration had seen an ongoing series of measures by the federal government aimed at constraining its outlays for Medicare, including the introduction of DRGs, physician fee controls, cutbacks in funding for capital and graduate medical education, the establishment of PRO-designated restrictions aimed at reducing unnecessary admissions and lengths of stay, and other interventions. Although the early results of many of these initiatives, particularly prospective hospital reimbursement, appear to be favorable, the long-term effectiveness of the new cost controls remains moot. Even if the DRG system falters, however, it is unlikely that cost-based reimbursement will be reinstated. We are much more likely to establish a new system of budgetary controls.

The last few years have called attention to the tenuousness of all long-term forecasts. In the early 1980s a potential deficit in the Medicare Trust Fund of $300 to $400 billion was widely posited. This prediction was no longer heard in 1987. Even in the face of continuing large deficits, Congress will avoid a radical reduction in Medicare benefits that would force the low-income elderly to contribute much more toward the cost of their hospitalization. It has moved to impose tax surcharges on the more affluent elderly, particularly for Medicare B coverage. If the federal budget goes totally out of control, it may be necessary to restructure Medicare into an essentially means-tested program.

Finally, the elderly must be more actively involved in the decisions affecting their health care and lives. Many states have acted, and others are likely to follow, to give the elderly or their responsible agents a larger role in deciding about life-support systems. The prolongation of life without independent function is not necessarily a boon. Death is not always the worse alternative.

Aging, and its concomitants, is a process that can prove unduly burdensome in an era in which many lack faith and others have little appreciation of fate. The elderly have need for understanding, reassurance, and support to help them bear the many infirmities for which there are no cures and at best only modest alleviation. A simple, straightforward book written for the elderly to help them through their declining years could be an invaluable resource, much as Dr. Spock's volumes on infant and child care were for the postwar generation of young mothers.

Concluding Observations

The extant system of funding health care for the elderly is fragile, and there is little or no prospect that the quantity and quality of care will be improved through substantially enlarged public expenditures in the near future. On the contrary, the current trend is toward constraints in both federal and state expenditures. However, in seeking to constrain public expenditures, care must be taken not to place excessive burdens on that half of the elderly population living on an annual income no greater than twice the poverty level. It should be a national imperative not to impose heavier burdens on those least able to bear them.

Some opportunities exist to reallocate resources. For example, reducing the quantity and intensity of acute hospital care utilized by the elderly (and others) would help finance the expansion of more appropriate and preferred services, such as home health care. It would be naive, however, to assume that such redirection of resources will come easily or quickly, given the power of the institutions and goals whose interest is to protect the status quo.

There is also little likelihood that potential improvements in the delivery of health-care services to the elderly will be realized unless the rapid inflation of health-care costs that has characterized the system during the past several decades can be slowed. The best prospect for moderating the anticipated steep increases in health-care services for the old-old, whose numbers are growing rapidly, rests with improvements in their health status through reduced morbidity, improved standards of living, and healthier lifestyles. If these improvements are reflected in fewer and lesser impairments in old age and if research and technology can modify the disabilities that are associated with dementia, incontinence, and immobility, our society will be better positioned to deal effectively and humanely with the health care needs of the elderly.

16

Psychiatry before the Year 2000

In the two decades after the end of World War II, much of my research was on the interface between the societal and psychological factors that determine effective or ineffective performance.[1] And in 1959 I was appointed to a four-year term on the advisory council of the National Institute of Mental Health (NIMH), then headed by Robert Felix. The years between 1945 and the mid-sixties saw the onset of the momentous changes in the use of drug therapy to treat mental disorders and the deinstitutionalization of the mentally ill.[2] During the last two decades and more, my research and policy roles have taken me into other domains, and therefore this present effort represents a new look at psychiatry, informed by old acquaintances and the additional perspective that comes with the passage of time.

Psychiatry in Camelot

During my years on the NIMH council in the early 1960s, I questioned four premises of the then current policy. It seemed to me, as a long-term specialist in manpower policy, that it was a questionable strategy to use federal funds to facilitate the retraining of primary care physicians and specialists as psychiatrists on the theory that by expanding the supply, the staff shortages in the state mental hospitals could be significantly alleviated.[3] I was not a fiscal conservative; I did not balk on the grounds that the use of federal funds for this purpose was inappropriate. Rather, I believed that the newly trained psychiatrists would not accept full-time or even part-time staff appointments in state hospitals but would establish private practices in urban centers, where they would treat the affluent.

My second disagreement with the director, his staff, and many of my colleagues on the council related to NIMH's steadily increasing requests for enlarged funding from Congress. Most of the new money was for research, but I doubted that the research that we were supporting held much promise of increasing our knowledge of the causes of mental illness or of developing new therapeutic leads to alleviate and cure such illness. I was depressed by the number and size of the grants that were approved for work in academic psychology, proposals that impressed the study sections. I warned Felix that as his budget grew from around $50 million to close to $200 million, Congress would soon start to ask some tough questions about the outcomes from its liberal appropriations.[4]

Several members of the NIMH staff had made recent visits to the United Kingdom and had been impressed by the progress that the British were achieving in treating large numbers of the mentally ill within the community instead of admitting them to distant hospitals. This cross-national experience contributed to the formulation and promotion of the community mental health center (CMHC) movement in the United States. Once again I was concerned. In my view, the federal government was not likely to provide long-term financing of such an effort; state support was problematic and, most important, the effective staffing of such centers would prove difficult. A modest demonstration effort seemed to be a sensible approach, but there was no sound basis for launching a national crusade.

In retrospect, it appears that the enthusiasm for CMHCs was the obverse of the effort to empty the state mental hospitals. The census in these hospitals had increased steadily until it peaked at about 560,000 in the mid-1950s. Efforts to treat more psychiatric patients in general hospitals, to improve treatment regimens in state hospitals, and to shift the site of continuing care for many patients from inpatient to outpatient settings were clearly desirable. But even rapid progress on each of these fronts was unlikely to empty the state mental hospitals. Our society has long required institutions of last resort for people who cannot care for themselves and need to be protected and maintained. The leaders of the reform failed to address the critical issue: if not state mental hospitals, then what?[5]

This review of psychiatric policy of the early 1960s provides a few useful lessons: enthusiasm is not a substitute for knowledge and understanding; a successful experiment is not a sufficient basis for developing a national program; ignoring the long-term realities of government operations, such as fashions in budgetary priorities, is certain prelude to failure and disaster; our existing knowledge and resources cannot eradicate the severe individual, family, and community disabilities stemming from mental illness; and the best we can hope to do is find ways to alleviate some of the burdens at a cost that society will continue to bear.

The Last Quarter-Century

Despite the shortfall between the ambitions and expenditures of the early 1960s and the realities of the 1980s, the last quarter of this century has seen important advances in psychiatry, particularly in the use of drug therapy for alleviating mental illness. Symptomatic relief in the absence of knowledge of the etiology of a disease must be considered a significant, not a minor, advance. Moreover, since the full adoption of a new technology is always attendant upon the education and training of a new generation of practitioners,[6] psycho-pharmacology holds promise of further gains in the years ahead.

On the clinical side, classical psychoanalysis has all but disappeared as a mode of treatment, largely because the potential patient group has concluded that the effectiveness of psychoanalytic therapy relative to its cost in time and money is problematic. Many have opted for treatment by other types of psychotherapists, particularly clinical psychologists and social workers, who offer more modest goals and lower fees but are not permitted to prescribe drugs. Most patients suffering from psychological disturbances with a somatic component continue to seek treatment from primary care physicians whose skills in diagnosing and treating such illness vary greatly.

Although psychiatrists bemoan the consequences of these patient flows, they have never succeeded in formulating practical alternatives for more effective triage. This challenge facing psychiatry has been complicated by a vast increase during the last decades in the number and proportion of patients seeking help for their emotional problems on an outpatient basis.[7]

Major changes have occurred in the distribution of psychiatric patients that reflect the belief that deinstitutionalization would lead to important gains in therapeutic outcomes and, further, would contribute to protecting the civil rights of individuals who were confined against their will.[8] But the policy of deinstitutionalization was primarily aided and abetted by developments in federal-state financing arrangements for Medicaid and Supplemental Security Income that created an overwhelming incentive for the states to push mental patients out of their institutions even if they required inpatient care. As long as inpatient care was provided in nursing homes or other settings to which the federal government contributed considerable funding, or that could use Social Security benefits for the elderly and the disabled to cover part of their maintenance costs, the burden on state budgets would be eased.

Although private insurance plans continued to discriminate against enrollees with psychiatric illnesses by providing less coverage for these illnesses and requiring higher copayments for their treatment, the expanded range and improved nature of health benefits contributed substantially to increasing the access of psychiatric patients to ambulatory and inpatient care in their communities.

All in all, mental health did not fare well in the competition for federal research dollars. The separation of the NIMH from the NIH and the formation of an expanded Alcohol, Drug Abuse, and Mental Health Administration that combined federal programs for mental health and alcohol and drug addiction helped to shift the focus away from research to education, demonstration projects, and program interventions. Fortunately, advances in molecular biology opened up some important research arenas in the neurosciences that received significant support from NIH.

In many large urban centers, such as New York City, deinstitutionalization led to the scandal of homeless street people, psychiatric patients who have been discharged from the hospital after a brief stay, with no alternative provision for their care and maintenance. Many of these patients are so severely disabled that they are a risk to themselves and on occasion to others. It has been estimated that between 1981 and 1985 New York City police transported about 63,000 such street people (some more than once) to a hospital for assessment, observation, and care. But within a few days or at most a few weeks these patients were discharged once again onto the streets.[9]

Despite the greater acceptance of mental illness as a fact of life and the larger numbers of Americans who seek treatment, the stigma that has been attached to mental illness and the skepticism about psychiatric treatment continue to color the beliefs of large numbers of patients, physicians, and payers. During the last decades, psychiatry has made some advances into the mainstream of American medicine, but so far it has not gained the full confidence of the voting and paying public.

The Changing Structure of Health Care

In the years to come, the likely developments in the health care sector will set bounds on the degrees of freedom that will be available to psychiatry. The two principal payers for health care—government and corporations—will continue to seek to contain the increases in their expenditures despite their lack of success to date.[10] Whether they succeed or not, they will redouble their efforts to moderate their outlays. Thus it is highly unlikely that the prevailing discrimination against psychiatric patients by Medicare and commercial insurance will be reduced or removed.

One trend, if it continues and strengthens, may redound to the advantage of psychiatry. Many large employers have become impressed with the cost-effectiveness of wellness programs. They are willing to make some investments in preventive medicine in the belief that reduced stress and less substance abuse will be reflected in less somatic illness as well as in less absenteeism and other dysfunctional patterns of work.

Following an ideological trend that predates the Reagan administration, state legislatures and the courts appear to be disinclined to support what they consider to be "monopolistic practices," which suggests for the case of psychiatry that qualified psychologists and social workers are likely to enjoy broader opportunities for independent practice, including independent billing.

Two recent developments run counter to the dominant trends of health care retrenchment. For one, it appears that the families of patients with mental illness have begun to step up their organizing activities to pressure state legislatures and Congress for relief from their burdens. The better organized advocacy groups are in a favorable position to lobby effectively so that at least in those states not in financial distress some new funding for improved mental health services should be forthcoming.

Moreover, there are signs that federal funding for research in psychiatry may be increased now that advocacy has been stepped up to educate the public and the Congress about the importance of enlarging the current level of support for psychiatric research. The pronounced shift toward managed care in the general health care market may result in an expanded demand for ambulatory mental health services. If payers and providers conclude that referrals to mental health practitioners can significantly reduce the numbers of "worried well" who clog the regular channels of care, they may become more willing to underwrite a reasonable volume of mental health services.

On the whole, however, current trends in the financing of health care are not likely to prove particularly beneficial to psychiatry. Rather, they suggest that psychiatry, like most of the house of medicine, will face a period of constrained resources that will make it difficult to broaden access to or to raise significantly the coverage and quality of existing services.

The Limits of Psychiatry

There are many different explanations for the reason psychiatry has remained in the antechamber of modern medicine. But one thesis that commands attention is the inherent contradiction between psychiatry as a field of specialization in the house of medicine and the claims advanced by its most articulate members, who regard the discipline as the answer to all forms of individual and social pathology, from the paranoid political leader to criminality and other social maladjustments. There is urgent need for the profession to consider the nature of its specialized knowledge and skills and the types of patients whom it can treat effectively even if it cannot cure many of them. Let's face it: many physicians treat patients whom they cannot cure. Psychiatrists have little to lose and much to gain by confronting and acknowledging this reality.

A related point is the radical shift during the last four decades to short-term therapy based on advances in drug therapy and the significant number of patients who receive symptomatic relief so that they can again function effectively. Psychiatry has no reason to be apologetic for the slow rate of its progress; it had earlier held exaggerated and, in terms of its knowledge base, unrealizable goals. The major afflictions of the mind—schizophrenia, affective disorders, senile dementia—like most of the cancers, are beyond the present knowledge and skill of the medical profession. Psychiatrists should acknowledge this fact and make it the centerpoint of their strategy. When physicians are unable to cure certain disorders, they must treat and seek to alleviate their patients' conditions. And they must redouble their efforts to encourage research so that more of the unknown becomes known. Research holds the greatest promise of eventually moving from alleviation to cure.

Psychiatry suffers from self-inflicted wounds. The mentally ill frequently are unable to function at minimum levels of competence because of their illnesses and thus they are the appropriate clientele of psychiatrists. But there are many other dysfunctional citizens in our society: the victims of inadequate schooling, racial discrimination, and unemployment, and others whose disabilities derive from the shortcomings of the society of which they are a part. These last victims may also suffer emotional scarring, but the roots of their malfunctioning are embedded in societal failures. Psychiatry can help itself, the victims of neglect, and the larger society by defining the scale and limits of its competence and by insisting that the body politic meet its responsibilities to its less fortunate citizens.

17

Medical Care for the Poor

At the time of the Great Society programs of President Johnson, many believed that with the passage of Medicare and Medicaid a single standard of superior medical care for all Americans was at hand. Governmentally funded entitlements for the elderly and the poor, the two major groups that lacked private health insurance, promised that limitations on access would soon be history. Clearly, that expectation has not been fulfilled. Rather, developments in the 1980s suggest that the numbers at risk because of lack of insurance coverage for health care are increasing. What lies back of the serious miscalculation?

In the mid-1980s estimates about the numbers of people who faced difficulties in obtaining medical care ranged from a low of 35 to 40 million persons who were without any form of insurance to roughly double that number if one includes all those not covered by major medical policies. But even the latter figure of 75 to 80 million, or 1 out of every 3 Americans, did not exhaust all who are at risk, since most major medical policies do not provide coverage for extended nursing home and home care services. Perhaps as many as half of all the elderly would be unprotected should they require care for an indefinite period; this would bring the total number at risk to close to 100 million or two out of five in the population.

The recent action of the Congress to amend Medicare by adding catastrophic coverage and the growing conviction among many leadership groups of the need to explore alternative mechanisms for financing long-term care point up one focus of current health policy debate. One must note, however, that even with catastrophic coverage for Medicare beneficiaries in place, patients requiring long-term care and patients with AIDS will still not be eligible for Medicare coverage.

Multiple efforts were under way in the mid-1980s to provide insurance coverage for those who currently lack it. In its Consolidated Omnibus Budget Reconciliation Act of 1985, Congress mandated that employers must offer discharged workers (and any dependents in the event of the worker's death) the option to convert at the group rate to an individual policy providing the same benefits; the duration of this coverage is 18 months for the employee and 36 months for survivors. Oregon took the lead to help small establishments provide insurance coverage for their employees through the use of subsidies. New York and New Jersey enacted categorical programs enabling groups with specific medical conditions to obtain coverage (New York's cystic fibrosis program and New Jersey's provisions for children with catastrophic illness are examples). In some states, Blue Cross continues to provide an open enrollment period using community rating for individuals and small groups. These various state efforts to extend the reach of insurance coverage to individuals and small employers face formidable impediments because of the progressive "fracturing" of the insurance pool: in an effort to reduce their costs, most large and many medium-sized employers had become self-insured. The cost of covering those previously excluded is just too high.

Another approach that was explored at both federal and state (Hawaii, California, and Massachusetts) levels was legislation requiring all employers to provide health insurance for their regular work force. A revised version of Governor Michael Dukakis's legislative proposal passed in Massachusetts, but Senator Edward Kennedy's comparable bill has yet to get through Congress.

Reform in the mid-1980s focused on federal and state efforts to broaden and deepen the Medicaid system by the introduction of greater flexibility, in particular loosening the link to welfare eligibility. Congress mandated transitional coverage for adults moving off welfare and coverage for all pregnant women and children under five years of age who met the financial criteria for Medicaid, whether or not they were recipients of Aid to Families with Dependent Children. In a radical move included in the Omnibus Budget Reconciliation Act of 1986, Congress permitted the states to set separate income standards for Medicaid eligibility and raise them to the federal poverty level (and higher) for pregnant women and children and also for the aged and disabled. By 1987 twenty-two states responded to the option.

Since the early 1980s, Congress has made it possible for the state Medicaid programs to experiment with new forms of service delivery to the poor through managed care programs that restrict the beneficiaries' freedom of choice in the selection of a personal physician. This is consonant with the belief of federal legislators and bureaucrats that one or another form of competition or managed care would result in both lower costs to the payers and better quality to the patients. With few exceptions, the states have not moved aggressively along this route, partly because of the opposition of the poor to loss of freedom of physician choice and the lack of cogent evidence that a Medicaid HMO or similar arrangement can in fact reduce the overall costs. Despite the widespread enthusiasm of many in and out of government about the efficacy of increased competition to control health care costs, they continue to increase.

The heavy concentration of the urban poor in specific neighborhoods and their long-term tendency to seek medical care from their community hospitals has resulted in burdening selected hospitals with the provision of disproportionate amounts of "charity care," that is, care for which they receive partial or no payment. Medicare takes this factor into account in calculating its DRG reimbursement schedules. A number of states have also established statewide financial pools which tax health insurance premiums or hospital revenues and redistribute the resultant funds to support hospitals that serve disproportionate numbers of nonpaying patients.

Attention should also be called to the extreme measure proposed in the state of Massachusetts to make participation in Medicaid a condition of physician licensure and refusal to treat a Medicaid patient cause for license revocation. The bill was withdrawn in favor of a voluntary agreement by the State Medical Society with the Medicaid program and this has significantly improved access of the poor to private physicians. In the case of Medicare, participating physicians are legally mandated to charge no more than the fee determined by HCFA for the services rendered, and violation is cause for license suspension or revocation.

Efforts to improve medical care for the poor must focus special attention on the Medicaid system as a whole and on public hospitals; these networks provide the financing and actual service delivery for the largest number of low-income individuals. Medicaid was set up as a federal-state system of personal medical care for the poor under which the federal government matches from 50 percent to 78 percent of the total program cost depending on the per capita income of the individual state. However, a considerable number of states, particularly in the South, had never appropriated sufficient sums to obtain the maximal federal contribution; as a result, annual Medicaid expenditures amounted to $951 per recipient in West Virginia and $993 in Mississippi as compared to $3,541 in New York and $3,675 in New Hampshire (1986 data).

In the same year more than 50 percent of all persons in the United States with incomes at or below the poverty line were *not* covered by Medicaid; eligibility cut-off ranged by state from as low as 25 percent of the poverty level to the federally established upper limit of 130 percent (except for special groups for whom the ceiling may be higher). Clearly, Medicaid is far from providing adequate coverage for the poor and even less for the near poor.

Nonfederal public hospitals accounted for 18 percent of all admissions for short-term care (1985 data). Many public hospitals, particularly those in large urban centers, operated at high levels of occupancy, 80 percent to 85 percent or above, frequently under conditions of inadequate professional staff, support personnel, and equipment. They are the providers of last resort and the principal source of hospital care for the urban poor. In rural areas, the poor who have no coverage are likely to face even greater difficulties in obtaining hospital care because of the shortage of public hospitals there.

Is the answer to the health problems of the poor that the United States should move expeditiously to introduce a federal or federal-state system of health insurance providing universal coverage? If the insurance pool continues to fracture and the economy moves further in the direction of small business, we may have no option but to replace the accidental linkage of health insurance and employment that was forged in World War II with a tax-based health insurance system. But it would be an error to assume that such a development would, by itself, effectively address the problems of medical care for the poor and the near poor. It would, to be sure, enable all persons to have access to ambulatory and in-patient care, but it would not specify the quantity and quality of such care. Beyond the elimination of the financial barrier, quantity and quality would continue to depend on the availability of physicians, support personnel, bed capacity, equipment, and other critical inputs. To take the argument one step further, without financial entitlement the poor will always be vulnerable. But removing the financial barriers to health care will at best alleviate, not solve, the problem.

We are a continental nation with vast regional and state differences in income, values, and standards of public services. Heretofore the federal government has never enforced a single standard of public service throughout the nation, whether in education, welfare, unemployment insurance, criminal justice, institutional care for the disabled and the mentally ill, or other social domains, including medical care. The only "equalizing" program that the federal government has enacted and successfully implemented has been the regular mailing of checks to Social Security beneficiaries.

The most reasonable expectation of action on the part of the federal government, budget permitting, is that it may be able to force or entice the states to shore up their Medicaid programs so that they can provide broader benefits to their poor and near poor. The heart of the challenge to the leadership lies in working toward a number of short and longer-term reforms that would improve access to medical services for the poor. We are not likely to see the quick establishment of a federal-state insurance system for all. The United States will have to undergo a long, and possibly bitter, political debate before reaching that goal. In the interim, we must try to improve the current, highly flawed situation, where lack of money often translates into lack of health care services.

In the near term there are things that we can and should do. In many states physician reimbursement for Medicaid patients is so low ($11 per visit in New York) that only a small minority of physicians, and surely not the best trained, treat them. Admittedly, many concerned and competent physicians continue to provide services for the poor without regard to the patient's ability to pay, but the number of poor who require inpatient and outpatient care far exceeds the philanthropic potential of physicians, hospitals, and nursing homes. It would be good public policy to redirect the flow of ambulatory Medicaid patients from hospital emergency rooms to private practitioners; to bring the per visit fee up to a reasonable level; and to use powerful professional and even governmental pressures to encourage physicians to treat greater numbers of the poor.

Similarly, a two-phased effort is required to reduce the concentration of the poor in public hospitals, even as these hospitals receive more resources to enable them to offer an acceptable level of care. With a surplus of acute care beds, there are opportunities in many communities to shift hospital care for the poor into mainstream institutions. And at the same time, it appears that the most effective short-term mechanism to facilitate this process would be federal and state reimbursement policies favoring hospitals that provide a large volume of charity care.

The thrust of my analysis has been to highlight the inherent limitations in a nonegalitarian society of continental proportions to establishing a single acceptable level of care for all its population and the inability to achieve this goal by passing more laws and appropriating more money, although some new laws and more money are definitely needed. The most important lessons, at least for the short-run, are these: more physicians must be encouraged (not coerced) to treat the poor and more of the poor need to be treated in mainstream community and teaching hospitals. Most important, the members of the medical profession must take the lead to persuade those who need to be persuaded at federal, state, and local levels that the ethic of medicine requires that all men and women have access to essential care, even if the wealthy are able to command and obtain more.

· V ·

Health
Agenda
Issues

18

Balancing Dollars and Quality

It is almost two decades since President Nixon warned the nation that the unremitting acceleration of health care costs threatened the stability of the U.S. economy. In 1970, the year that the president declared a crisis in health care, total expenditures amounted to $75 billion or 7.5 percent of GNP. The figures for 1989 indicate outlays of over $620 billion or more than 11.2 percent of GNP. Clearly, President Nixon was prematurely concerned about the level of health care outlays and their dangers to the well-being of the U.S. economy. Ever since President Nixon first sounded the alarm, we have heard from different quarters—businessmen, academics, politicians—that the nation cannot continue to spend an ever larger portion of its GNP on health care. Many in recent years have suggested an upper limit of 10 percent of GNP.

There are a number of reasons to question this judgment. Uwe Reinhardt has repeatedly pointed out that the amounts spent for health care appear on the revenue side of the national accounts as income—for physicians, nurses, a wide variety of health workers, the pharmaceutical industry, and many others who provide intermediate or final goods and services to the health sector. Indeed, health care is the nation's third largest source of employment—following only government and retailing. About 1 out of every 13 members of the labor force is employed in the health sector.

Although I have questioned the conventional wisdom that we cannot afford to spend an ever larger proportion of our national income on health care, I do not want to leave the impression that there is no upper limit to such outlays. As of 1988, however, I see no reason why expenditures should not rise to 15 percent or possibly as much as 20 percent of our GNP.

True, we must be able to sell abroad American goods and services to cover our imports of both merchandise and capital or at least the interest payments on our foreign borrowings. Health care, by and large, does not contribute to this task. We should, however, be able to accumulate sufficient revenues from our export trade to pay for our imports even if our health care expenditures reach the 15 to 20 percent level of GNP.

A related point: we are a democracy that relies heavily on consumer sovereignty. This means that politicians are willing to spend large sums only when they get clear signals from their constituents. At present, government at all levels is spending approximately $250 billion for health care. The employer community commits somewhat under $185 billion for health insurance benefits for employees, an outlay that reflects the preferences of most workers, if not all. The remaining $185 billion represents direct out-of-pocket payment by consumers.

I am hard-pressed to read the evidence as anything other than an expression of the American people's willingness to spend $500 billion annually on health care. Nobody is coercing them to do so; it reflects their preference. Of course, most Americans would like to obtain their present quantity and quality of care at a lower cost but since that has not proved feasible, they are willing to absorb the higher bill. In fact, most opinion polls indicate the widespread desire of the public for still more health care services although they are ambivalent as to how the increment is to be paid for.

As an observer of the changing U.S. health care scene since the 1930s, I have been impressed with the dramatic rise in the quality of health care in the U.S. (and in other advanced countries) even as the dollars consumed by the health care sector have increased simultaneously by orders of magnitude. Some economists, led by Alain Enthoven of Stanford University, have called attention to what is termed the "flat of the curve," an economist's abstraction which suggests that with additional dollars of expenditure there are no commensurate increases in productive outcomes. The concept is sound. However, modern medicine requires the passage of many years before it can be determined whether or not a specific expenditure is justified. In the early days of the new imaging technology, Kerr White was critical of the widespread introduction of the CAT scanner, arguing that it would be used for every patient who complained of headache. Some, possibly many, patients undergo unnecessary CAT scans, unnecessary at least if the findings are negative. But that is a naive criterion. One of the great potentialities of quality medicine is the ability to rule out the presence of serious pathology.

Quality Health Care

From the perspective of a patient, quality health care may be defined as an ongoing relationship with a well-trained physician whose knowledge and judgment I trust, who is competent to treat me himself or will refer me for whatever other health care services I may require. It further implies that I have adequate insurance coverage to pay for the range of services that the physician(s) believe will contribute optimally to my recovery without exposing me to undue risks. Since I am convinced that the patient must play an active role in his treatment and recovery, another important dimension of quality health care is the ability and willingness of the physician to communicate effectively with me on all aspects of my treatment about which I need to be apprised. I must also be self-motivated or encouraged by my physician to adopt a sensible regimen.

One further aspect of quality medical care is frequently overlooked, though less so than in years past. Medicine is part science, part art and individuals differ in their goals and risk-taking behavior. Therefore, a competent physician must lay out for his patient the risk-benefit ratios that attach to alternative forms of intervention, or the choice of no intervention at all. To an avid tennis-player, submitting to an orthopedic operation of uncertain outcome may make sense. A sedentary individual might avoid the possibly negative outcome by deciding to forego the operation.

Contributors to Quality Care

Medical educators, by establishing a high standard of medical education, have contributed greatly to assuring the competence of American physicians. The specialty societies through their residency review committees and their certification procedures have likewise had a significant effect. In partnership with them, the academic health centers and the major teaching hospitals have set and pursued high standards of care which have served as a model that most community hospitals have sought to emulate.

The large-scale financial support of the federal government for biomedical research, currently in excess of $7 billion annually, has contributed to scientific and technical advances across many fronts. Likewise, small and large companies, particularly in the pharmaceutical industry and in the fields of medical equipment and supplies, have been responsible for many technological breakthroughs. At the same time, the regulatory powers of the FDA have protected the American consumer from many harmful drugs and appliances (though at the cost of delaying access to beneficial new products).

Labor-management support for private health insurance has provided the essential financial coverage, without which quality health care would have been unobtainable for most Americans. Federal financing for Medicare and federal-state financing for Medicaid have provided good access for the elderly to quality acute care, inpatient and ambulatory. However, the opportunities that were made available to the poor were for the most part badly designed and did not enable them to obtain treatment by the best physicians or in superior hospitals.

While the leaders of the medical profession have decried the proliferation of malpractice suits, contending that this has necessitated the practice of "defensive" medicine—that is, the performance of more tests and more procedures than would be justified for optimal medical care—I would argue that increasing recourse to the courts has, on balance, probably resulted in more conscientious, considered physician practice and thereby contributed to the quality of care that patients receive.

The rising level of general education of the public (whose formal education, on average, now extends beyond high school graduation) has undoubtedly enhanced their sophistication in dealing with personal medical problems, both with respect to the selection of a physician and other choices that they must make. The substantial and sustained interest of the media, despite periodic distortions and exaggerations about new therapies and cures, has also contributed to making the public more sophisticated consumers of health care. More education and better media coverage of health affairs must be viewed as contributions to increasing quality.

One of the most potent agents of quality improvement has been the complex of rules and regulations that now govern the operations of acute care hospitals; these include the process of staff selection, the scheduling of clinical pathological conferences, grand rounds, special lectures, and informal consultations among staff members. Closely related to the foregoing is the elaborate structure of continuing educational opportunities sponsored by diverse medical leadership groups, ranging from the development of cassettes for the physician to listen to while driving in the car, to a wide array of meetings and clinical conferences, which tend to be well attended. In a field such as medicine, where new knowledge and new techniques are constantly emerging, broad exposure to the most recent developments is essential if the existing practitioner group is not to be left behind.

Finally, reference must be made to the sizable licensing and control apparatus that is vested in local, state, and federal governmental agencies, and in a variety of nonprofit agencies. Beginning with initial licensing and certification, they conduct extensive audit and control functions, such as mandatory institutional reporting, comparative analysis of operating information, and publication of the performance records of individual hospitals. While there have been serious complaints about the multiplicity of these control instruments, their duplication, and poor follow-up (if any), on balance one might see them as contributions, however imperfect, to raising the quality of care. Except for Milton Friedman and a small number of extremist libertarians who consider the licensing of physicians unnecessary and unworkable, few would argue in favor of discarding the effort entirely.

Responsibility for quality care is thus widely diffused, resting in the first instance with the various leadership groups in the health care profession, and extending to a complex network involving governmental agencies, the public, and the media.

What Are the Ethical Issues?

The medical profession has not directly confronted the issue of how to determine, under conditions of constant change, the criteria for the specification of "an essential level of care" that should be available to all persons. Failing such a definition and failing the commitment by the medical leadership of its substantial prestige to assure that this standard is universally applied, large numbers of individuals will as the result of lack of money, ignorance, and other barriers be exposed to an inferior quality of care.

In fact, the medical leadership has found it difficult to establish an effective mechanism by which to fulfill its responsibility to the state, which has granted it wide discretion in the use of self-regulation to maintain oversight of the profession and to discipline members who for reasons of health, competence, or behavior, are a threat to their patients. The AMA has estimated the number of "impaired" physicians to be between 5 and 10 percent; nevertheless, except in the most egregious instances— and usually after serious harm has been done—the profession and the licensing authorities have taken virtually no action. The medical profession has found it very difficult, perhaps impossible, to be an effective policeman. Hence the public remains at considerable risk as a result of the inability of the profession to establish an effective system of control, which requires close cooperation with public authorities.

The science and art of medicine are practiced within the framework of a societal value system which has legal, religious, ethical and other parameters that intersect with health care decision-making and action. The Baby Doe case exemplifies one such intersection; the Brophy case (the removal of a feeding tube from a patient in a permanent vegetative state) another. There are many more; witness the large numbers of Americans who have signed living wills to assure that they will not be subjected to heroic interventions in the event that they are judged incapable of regaining reasonable functionality.

Since people differ in their views about life and death and the states in-between, the courts have placed heavy weight on the autonomy of the patient to accept or reject treatment; when the patient is not competent to make such a judgment his next of kin are authorized to decide for him or her. It is generally agreed that medical decisions are best made in hospitals, not in the courtroom, and an increasing number of hospitals have established medical ethics committees to provide guidelines for patients' families and the hospital staff in determining how to proceed in borderline situations. The discipline of medical ethics has undergone steady elaboration in recent years, and this is reflected in its representation in the curriculum and faculty of medical schools, and the establishment of journals, centers, and related institutions dedicated to probing and clarifying the changing relations between medicine and these critical value areas.

The United States has thus far been reluctant to face up to the inherent dilemmas of certain new technologies such as the allocation of organs for transplant when the number of available organs is far short of the number of potential beneficiaries. The institutions that perform heart, liver, and kidney transplants have for the most part established their own criteria for the selection of recipients; here the ability to pay has loomed large even when it has not been the ultimate determinant.

A more subtle aspect of the dollar-quality tension is revealed by the submerged but nonetheless real competition for expensive care among different age cohorts in the population, particularly between the young and the old. Medicare provides substantial funding for the acute health care of persons over 65 and for the permanently disabled between the ages of 55 and 65. But there is no comparable source of funding for the young except via the Medicaid mechanism, which is a much more limited source of support. Some people feel strongly that it is a violation of both ethics and good sense for a society to deflect so much of its resources to the care of the elderly nearing the end of their days while depriving the young, whose lives are still before them, of needed therapeutic and rehabilitative care. The competition among these age groups for funding appears to be grounded in the greater "political leverage" of the elderly who are active, voluble voters, while youth have only their parents to lobby for them.

In the early 1970s Congress decided to make all persons suffering from end-stage kidney disease eligible for federally funded (Medicare) renal dialysis. Since then it has refused, for financial reasons, to single out any other disease category for similar consideration, including AIDS, although in that case the period between definitive diagnosis and death has not been longer than two years. It would be hard to fault the Congress for having acted as it did in the case of renal dialysis or for having refused to act similarly with respect to other disease categories.

Another complex ethical issue in the dollar-quality arena relates to the values that are expressed in keeping extremely immature neonates alive even in the face of a high probability that they will be doomed to a life of severe disability which for many, if not all, will require continuing institutionalization or special care and impose heavy burdens on their parents and other children in the household. Admittedly, great strides have been made in saving underweight newborns but the question remains: what constraints, if any, should be placed on the efforts of researchers and clinicians to save infants of ever smaller birthweight?

Still another ethical issue relates to the decision-making of a society that spends, on the average, $2,000 per capita every year for the health care of its members and ignores the substantial increase in the number of children being reared in poverty and their needs. Two fifths of all young families with children had incomes at or below half of the poverty level in 1986. Once again, it is difficult in seeking an explanation to overlook the relative voting strengths of the two competing groups, the middle class and the poor.

We have identified seven categories of ethical issues that intersect with questions of the quality of medical care, specifically:

- Access of all to essential care.

- The control of impaired physicians.

- Decisions affecting high-tech interventions in the face of poor prospects of quality life.

- The rationing of organ transplants.

- Inequalities in medical care available to youth and the elderly.

- Preferential treatment for victims of kidney disease under Medicare.

- The proportionate allocation of public monies between

health and other critical needs (such as income maintenance for the poor).

These seven illustrations are a potent reminder that ethical issues are embedded in all aspects of our health care system even
though many of them remain hidden from view.

Some Practical Steps for Improvements

If ours were not a resource-constrained society and all individuals had access to quality medical care, there would still be
ethical issues confronting the polity. Nowhere is that more clear
than in the area of living wills, to which many educated and
affluent persons increasing resort to protect themselves against
excessive medical treatment when restoration to a state of reasonable functionality is unlikely. This reevaluation of the right
to life has gone even further in the Netherlands, where under
strict professional and legal control euthanasia is countenanced.

Our ethical problems in the health arena are closely linked to
the fact that we are a society that favors unequal distribution of
income and capital even as it professes that all persons should,
in times of need, have access to medical care. Moreover, it is a
society that seeks to avoid imposing heavy tax burdens on the
citizenry and this tends to restrict the flow of public dollars into
the health arena. This resistance to large public spending for
health has manifested itself much more in the case of the poor
and children than in the case of the elderly. A first challenge,
therefore, is to see to it that our imperfect Medicaid structure,
the major program for providing access to the poor, is considerably strengthened. Fortunately, Congress has mandated in recent
years that the states provide broader coverage for women and
children. In many other areas, however, Congress has been loath
to set minimum standards and a considerable number of states
have consistently failed to appropriate sufficient funds to take
full advantage of the maximum (78 percent) contribution of the
federal government.

It is not easy in our federal-state system of governance, with
large variations in economic potential, racial composition, values, and public services, to establish a reasonable minimum
standard of care for the poor that would encompass meaningfully

both Mississippi and New York—but that is the first challenge that we face. As indicated earlier, the medical profession must play a part, in fact a leading part, in determining within each state what should be an essential level of care to be provided to all its residents. Without the active participation of the medical profession, satisfactory standards cannot be established and will not be enforced.

There is increasing concern, especially among the elderly, that our society must respond to the challenge of long-term care, to which Medicaid currently devotes about 40 percent of its total expenditures. The fundamental question is not whether we should experiment with new and better ways to provide health coverage and services to the sick and frail elderly, but rather whether the very large task of long-term care should be interpreted primarily as a medical or a social challenge. With a very few exceptions—notably senile dementia, deteriorative neurological diseases, and incontinence where institutionalization may be the preferred or only alternative—I believe that most of the problems of the feeble elderly are primarily in the nature of social rather than medical support. They and their families need help to care for them at home.

There is a related issue of the 40 million or more persons who lack health insurance. Most of them are not poor and most of them are employed; in the event of a serious illness, however, they would be at serious risk in obtaining access to quality care. The country is experimenting with various devices, among them mandated health benefits by all employers, state risk pools to enable small employers to purchase coverage at an affordable cost, and state surcharges on hospital revenues that are redistributed among institutions that provide differential amounts of charity care.

It remains to be seen whether any of these efforts will solve the problem. I doubt it. My guess is that the number of uncovered individuals will continue to increase. Some believe that the only sensible approach for the United States is to follow the pattern of all other advanced countries and adopt a federal or federal-state system of health insurance. The proposal has much to commend it but in light of the inherent difficulties arising from state variations in economic resources and social values it is hard to conceive of a national system that would be equally responsive to rich and poor states alike. And it cannot be assumed that the program would be sufficiently funded over time to avoid the imposition of widespread rationing; this has been the experience of every country that has adopted a system of national health insurance.

National health insurance aside, the American people must devote attention and effort to questions of rationing which are inherent in high-tech medicine, particularly in the arena of transplants. We may be able to ignore the complex issues that rationing precipitates for a while longer, but only if we believe that avoidance is preferable to analysis and consensual decision-making. The medical ethicists must play an important role in clarifying the many complications involved in the determination of who should live and who must die.

The several instances discussed thus far have revealed the implicit, if not explicit, struggle over resources within the health care sector and between the health care sector and other public goods such as welfare and education, struggles that pit the elderly against youth, and these surely warrant the attention of the public. In guiding the debate both ethicists and economists have important roles to play in sharpening the issues and evaluating the evidence required for improved decision-making. Incidentally, it does not follow that if the public decides to be less generous in the money it provides for the health care of the elderly, it would necessarily appropriate the "saved" sums for education or welfare. The odds are that it would not.

We are a considerable distance from affording every American access to quality medical care, or even to essential medical care. However, the nation did make great gains toward achieving these goals in the post-World War II era. In moving in this direction, the United States increased its expenditures about sevenfold in constant dollars, fivefold on a per capita basis. The HCFA estimates that our current level of spending is likely to double within seven years and triple within twelve years. If our economy does not falter, the probabilities are good that the forecast will turn out to be within the ballpark.

Despite such substantial outlays, I suspect that the proportion of the population that will lack access to quality care will not be significantly different than it is at present. The reason, as I have emphasized, is that we have no readily available mechanism to establish and enforce national standards for the provision of any set of combined public and private services throughout this large and diversified nation. Moreover, our efforts will focus more on advancing the accomplishments of high-tech medicine and diffusing its benefits broadly than on assuring equality of access.

However, we have long been a people whose individualism and entrepreneurship have been moderated by a heavy dose of religiosity and compassion so that we have not turned our back on those who have fallen behind in the struggle for services. It is essential that the medical ethicists, among others, continue to goad the conscience of the public so that it acts to insure that all of the polity have access to essential care.

19

A Hard Look at Cost Containment

This chapter addresses three interrelated questions: What does the record reveal about the success of two decades of efforts at cost containment? What lessons can be extracted from this experience? What is the outlook for cost containment in the middle and longer term?

Because the United States population grew rapidly over this quarter century and the economy was buffeted by inflationary pressures, the best single index of expenditures is the per capita outlay in constant dollars, which shows a gain of 133 percent. The percentage of the GNP contributed by health care expenditures in the period 1960–1985 reveals that economic growth supplied only part of the additional resources that were needed to cover increases in health care costs.

The data underscore that health expenditures in the United States have been increasing rapidly; they have accounted for a steadily rising share of the GNP; and the steepest rate of increase (in constant dollars) occurred in the five years after the introduction of Medicare and Medicaid in 1965.

The Cost Containment Record

Throughout the 1970s, the federal government and many of the states sought to contain health care costs through planning, regulation, and controls on hospital costs. In the waning days of the Carter administration, however, Congress balked at continuing on the regulatory route and rejected the president's proposal to impose an annual ceiling on capital expenditures for new hospital construction.

The Reagan administration entered office with a strong anti-regulation bias and looked to enlarging the scope of the market and price competition to control health care costs.[1] But it failed to develop a comprehensive strategy aimed at deregulating health care. New competitive forces and a broadened role for price competition have increasingly come to characterize health care, however. Four specific developments are viewed as the foundations of cost containment: the introduction of prospective financing for Medicare beneficiaries who require hospitalization, the proliferation of new forms of prepaid health care delivery, the increasing supply of physicians, and the growth of for-profit health care enterprises.

In assessing the success or failure of cost-containment efforts, it is essential to consider the total use of resources in relation to total useful output, measured by quality as well as quantity. Cost containment should not be confused with cost shifting or with cost reductions in one area, such as inpatient care, without taking into account cost increases in another, such as ambulatory treatment. True cost containment depends on controlling the costs of the health care system as a whole, without impairing quality.[2]

Hospital admissions and days of care peaked before the introduction of diagnosis-related groups in 1983; nevertheless, the federal government's shift to prospective reimbursement for hospital care for Medicare patients unquestionably accelerated the trend toward reducing the number of inpatient hospital days.[3] Since expenditures on hospital care account for 40 percent of total health care outlays, many have interpreted fewer admissions and shorter stays as major contributions to cost containment, especially because the growth of managed care systems and the expanding scope of ambulatory treatment are seen as further opportunities to reduce overall hospital days.

William B. Schwartz has recently challenged this optimistic view.[4] He has pointed out that the current reductions reflect a one-time gain that results from removing the "fat" in the hospital system and that the underlying factors—continuing advances in technology, population growth, and rising prices (particularly more expensive labor)—will reverse the initial decline in the rate of growth of health care costs and maintain an increase in costs of about 7 percent a year. I agree with the thrust of his analysis. Moreover, the cost per hospital admission has continued to increase, even as some of the fat has been removed;[5] despite severe reductions in occupancy, downscaling and closings of hospitals have been proceeding at a snail's pace,[6] and most calculations of cost containment in inpatient treatment fail to take into account new expenditures for ambulatory care, nursing home services, and home care.

The rapid growth of enrollments in HMOs and PPOs is perceived as the necessary precursor of effective cost containment.[7] Admittedly, HMO enrollees have a much lower rate of hospitalization than patients under traditional fee for service. But several important countervailing factors need to be considered. HMO and fee-for-service costs have been found to grow at the same rate.[8] Despite the recent rapid growth of prepaid plans, not more than one in six Americans was covered by an HMO or a PPO at the beginning of 1987. The assumption that at least two of every five insured persons will be enrolled in a prepaid plan by the 1990s is probably too optimistic in the face of the steeply growing costs of marketing, the absence of large savings to employers, the difficulties of structuring and managing large prepaid plans, and the growing insistence of employers and consumers on quality controls. The continuing, if somewhat slower, growth of prepaid health plans can be expected to exercise some restraint on cost increases, but it will not be sufficient to reverse their upward trend.

Between 1970 and 1986, the number of physicians per 100,000 population increased from 148 to 220. During the same years, the net pretax income of physicians, in constant dollars, averaged $35,942 (1970) and $35,133 (1985).[9] Applying supply-and-demand analysis to physician services, most mainline economists have looked favorably on increases in the supply of physicians in the expectation that this increase would lower physicians' fee schedules and earnings. The income data just mentioned provide little support for such a conclusion. In most market areas and in most fields of specialization, established physicians are able to influence both the demand for their services (by encouraging return visits by their patients) and their incomes (by raising their fees).[10]

Further increases in the supply of physicians are inevitable because of the large numbers of students already being trained. Even if a further increase of 20 percent in the supply of physicians would depress physicians' earnings by 20 percent, total health care costs would be much more likely to increase than to decline. Since physicians' earnings account for about 20 percent of total health care expenditures, the savings realized from a reduction in physicians' incomes would be 4 percent. Physicians are said, however, to be responsible for 70 percent of total health care outlays. Hence, a 20 percent increase in their number would generate an increased outlay of 14 percent, or a net increase in health care expenditures of 10 percent. Because most of the physical facilities of the health care system are now in place, it would be reasonable to reduce this estimate of the additional costs of the new supply of physicians by half—that is, from 10 to 5 percent. But with expenditures now in excess of $500 billion, even the incremental costs of the additional physicians would be substantial, adding $25 billion annually.

The emergence and rapid growth of for-profit hospital chains in the 1970s and the more recent incursion of for-profit enterprises into other areas of health care are viewed by many as the harbingers of greater cost effectiveness resulting from economies of scale, equity financing, and professional management. Some advocates have gone so far as to prophesy that a dozen or so large for-profit health care companies will soon come to dominate the entire health care sector.[11]

There is no reliable evidence that for-profit hospitals provide equivalent care for less money than nonprofit hospitals.[12] R. E. Herzlinger and W. S. Krasker argued that in view of the tax subsidies to nonprofit hospitals, the lower cost at which they are able to borrow money, and the undermaintenance of their plants, the for-profit hospitals have the edge.[13] However, their inquiry is restricted to a very short period of rapid hospital growth (1977 through 1981), and their sample included only 3 percent of all nonprofit hospitals but half of all for-profit hospitals. Furthermore, many nonprofit hospitals provide unique societal services such as education and research, which the for-profit hospitals do not provide. These caveats limit the value of their contribution to health policy.

Even Wall Street has become much less bullish on the for-profit hospital chains; several of the chains have moved from a policy of acquisition to selling off some hospitals that do not fit their new strategies, and their occupancy rates are many points below those of the nonprofit hospitals—a fact that does not augur well for their balance sheets in the future. Only a true believer in private enterprise and the competitive market will look to the for-profit chains for the solution to the problem of the nation's rising health care expenditures.

The boundaries of medicine are continually being expanded, as demonstrated by the new programs for sports medicine, cosmetic surgery, wellness, substance control, and health education—not to mention the uncertainties that attach to the spread of AIDS. Although hospital capacity may eventually be considerably reduced, alternative forms of care are likely to proliferate. And the number of physicians—the key determiners of the use of health care resources—will increase. All these point to cost increases, not cost containment.

The Middle- and Longer-Term Outlook

In the period from 1985 to 1990 health care expenditures increased by 8.4 percent, the lowest increase in any five-year period since the effort at cost containment was first launched. Yet the cost spiral continues. Why does it, and what forces might sooner or later interrupt or possibly even reverse it?

The first question is relatively easy to answer: costs rise because we permit them to rise. Our "open system" of health care has numerous sources of funding. The federal government, the largest payer, covers only about one third of the total bill. Corporations, through their benefit plans, cover something over one quarter. The remaining major payers are consumers (who pay out of pocket), states, and other levels of government. With more than 30 million of the nation's elderly persons holding paid membership in the AARP, Congress will find it difficult, if not impossible, in the absence of an overriding financial crisis, to cut back substantially on Medicare benefits.

State governments are wrestling with the urgent need to improve their Medicaid programs and are exploring alternative ways to protect the uninsured through subsidized insurance or a mechanism for reimbursing providers who care for the insured. Many corporations have been successful in recent years in renegotiating health care benefits for their employees, with the result that employees now have less first-day coverage and pay more out of pocket for health care in the form of deductibles and coinsurance. Costs rise in one sector and recede in another, but the system as a whole depends on the decisions of the federal and state legislatures, large and medium-sized corporations, and consumers. The American people have indicated repeatedly, in response to surveys, that they want more and better health care services.[14] And many nonprofit, for-profit, and government health care providers are able to continue to enter the capital markets and obtain new funding to meet these increased demands.

What about the longer term? Clearly, there is an upper limit on the proportion of the GNP that the American people will be willing to spend on health care—possibly 15 percent, perhaps as much as 20 percent. But before we reach that theoretical upper limit, other forces may come into play. We could face a major crisis in the federal budget, which could lead to the transformation of Medicare into a means-tested program. We could fail to provide essential care to increasing numbers of uninsured persons, thereby creating renewed political momentum for national health insurance. The competitive position of American business could become so endangered that a growing number of large, medium-sized, and small corporations would have no alternative but to cut back on employees' health care benefits. One can think of other pressures and responses, including limiting the introduction of high-cost technology and explicit attempts to ration high-cost treatments.

A society such as ours—which places a high value on pluralism, which is enthralled by technology, which resists domination by the federal government, which accepts the prevailing inequality of income and wealth, and which promotes the sovereignty of consumers—is not likely to opt for serious constraints on biomedical research and development or to favor the explicit rationing of proved health care services to the public. Its concerns are more likely to be focused on ensuring access for the entire population to an effective level of care and on finding a way of covering the health care costs of those who cannot pay their own way. Until we approach the upper limit of acceptable health care expenditures—an eventuality that may be far in the future—cost containment is likely to remain the elusive hare that the hounds pursue but never overtake.

20

U.S. Health Policy:
Expectations and Realities

The year 1988 was a good time to take stock of U.S. health policy. Twenty-five years ago the federal government acted vigorously to expand the number of medical school graduates by an order of magnitude; twenty years ago the Congress first became aware that the costs of Medicare would far exceed the original estimates and, accordingly, eliminated the 2 percent override in reimbursements to hospitals. And 1988 saw the first significant increase in Medicare entitlements when President Reagan signed into law the catastrophic insurance bill.

This longer retrospective emphasizes the extent to which earlier expectations have been fulfilled or, alternatively, undermined by later events. The increase of more than 60 percent in the ratio of physicians to population, from 140 to 233 per 100,000 (1960 to 1988),[1] failed to ensure that all patients would have ready access to a physician; nevertheless, the expanded supply surely eased the problem of access. Medicare met its goal of enabling most of the elderly to obtain acute care without financial stress, but it fell far short of providing for their total health care needs, particularly the need for long-term care. Medicaid enabled the eligible poor to obtain improved access to the health care system; nevertheless, it did not lead to the establishment of a single level of care for all Americans. Less than half of the population living in poverty was covered by Medicaid in 1988; about 40 million persons were not covered and another 40 million had shallow coverage. While the last quarter century saw a broadening and deepening of the US health care system, 1988 found the nation with many unsolved problems on its health policy agenda and a profusion of scenarios for reform based more on theory than fact. It is difficult for a democracy to solve problems about which a consensus exists; it is next to impossible for it to do so if it is loaded down with beliefs that run counter to reality. We will examine briefly ten policy areas that fall into that category.

Cost Containment. The three largest payers for health care—the federal government (30 percent of total national expenditures), state and local governments (10 percent), and employers (30 percent)[2]—have been engaged with varying degrees of intensity in slowing their outlays for health care. Government has resorted to subsidizing the formation of new forms of health care provision, reducing the number of persons eligible to receive services, and adopting a system of prospective reimbursement for the hospitalization of Medicare patients (DRGs). And employers have opted to self-insure and renegotiate employee health care benefits to shift more of the costs of care onto the beneficiaries.

All of the talk and action notwithstanding, the data provide unequivocal evidence that cost containment has been largely sound and fury signifying little. Between 1970 and 1987 total outlays rose from $75 billion to $497 billion, or from 7.5 percent of the gross national product (GNP) to 11.2 percent.[3]

Wasteful and Ineffective Care. A number of sophisticated health care analysts, notably the former Secretary of Health, Education, and Welfare, Joseph Califano,[4] and Robert Brook[5] and John Wennberg[6] have called attention to the "waste" in the system of medical care exemplified in physicians' doing too much and, worse still, often performing diagnostic and therapeutic procedures that are contraindicated in the opinion of the leaders of the profession. With half a million physicians active in patient care, who have different training and practice in different localities, it is not surprising that controlled studies confirm many questionable diagnostic and therapeutic practices. Thus far, however, the investigators and the critics have failed to design a practical program for identifying and eliminating the suspect and harmful interventions.

Neither the profession nor the public would be well served by nationally imposed norms of practice, however. Unless physicians and patients are willing to experiment with the new, medical practice will stagnate. Old drugs and old procedures are constantly being reassessed and discarded through an extensive learning network, from medical conferences to vast medical literature. It is not clear how the presumed widespread waste could be effectively eliminated except at a cost in excess of the benefits.

Physician supply. In 1976, thirteen years after the federal government became the lead party in expanding the nation's physician supply, Congress declared that the physician shortage was at an end. In 1980 the GMENAC reported the findings of its four-year study, alerting the nation that it would face a serious surplus of physicians in 1990 and a larger surplus in the year 2000. Six years later, in 1986, the House of Delegates of the AMA reversed its long-held position that the market was the best regulator of physician supply and warned of the coming surplus and the need for corrective action. But in the spring of 1988 the prestigious *New England Journal of Medicine* published two articles by competent analysts who argued from the data that there was little prospect of a surplus by the year 2000 and more likely a shortage after 2010, when the baby boomers will reach retirement age.[7]

In no way can recourse to statistical calculations alone determine whether the nation faces a surplus, a balance, or a shortage of physicians some years in the future. The answer must be sought in the context of the following issues: How much money will the public be willing to spend in the future on medical care? What are the margins for substituting other health professionals for physicians? What is the appropriate patient load for a specialist to carry to ensure the maintenance of his skills? How serious is the danger to the public of overtreatment by physicians with unfilled appointment books?

Health Maintenance Organizations. In 1973 Congress decided to make federal funding available to facilitate the establishment of new HMOs and the expansion of existing ones, in the belief that they could reduce the costs of providing health care services. Despite these subsidies, HMOs experienced desultory growth until the early 1980s, when many employers got behind them and encouraged their workers to sign up. The result was a rapid spurt in HMO enrollments, although as of the end of 1987 the figure had reached just 29.3 million, no more than 12 percent of the population.[8]

Little attention has been given to the fact that most of the new HMOs were for-profit organizations that did not conform to the classic staff model (group practice, with physicians being paid on a per capita basis) but relied instead on Individual or Independent Practice Associations. More important, the tightening of admissions and length of stay in acute care hospitals reduced, if it has not yet eliminated, the principal competitive advantage of HMOs over fee-for-service medicine. And not enough attention has been paid to the growing signs of economic distress among HMOs: more than two out of three failed to earn a profit in 1986.

The Pro-Competition Solution. In the second half of the 1970s, President Carter sought to introduce legislation authorizing the federal government to limit the total amount of new capital that could be invested annually in acute care hospitals. His advisers believed that this was the best way to slow the steep acceleration in hospital expenditures. After a bruising fight between the administration and an array of interests spearheaded by the AHA, the bill was defeated twice. The hospital industry and the Congress had reached the conclusion that more regulation was not the way to go.

Alain Enthoven,[9] author of the "pro-competition" approach, proposed that the purchasers of insurance be encouraged to shop around on the basis of price among multiple health care provision systems, which he believed would emerge in a competitive environment. Although the Carter administration was never convinced of the Enthoven proposal, the Reagan administration heralded it as the mechanism to slow cost acceleration and to reduce the heavy hand of government. Ironically, the major Reagan cost-containment initiative—prospective reimbursement for hospital expenditures on behalf of Medicare beneficiaries—turned out to be, as Alan Greenspan has noted, nothing other than a governmental price-fixing scheme, light years away from a competitive system.

Private Insurance. Health analysts have generally failed to note the paradox that most large- and medium-sized corporations—the flagships of our competitive economy—overlooked the upward creep of their health care expenditures until the severe depression of 1981. At that point they made a series of moves; not the least important of these was to opt for self-insurance and to rely on their former underwriters simply for administrative support. They considered it advantageous to insure their own employees rather than continue to be part of a larger pool that was likely to contain a greater number of high-risk individuals. Although this presumption was valid, self-insurance was not sufficient to brake the rise in their total health care costs. A development they failed to appreciate and that has only recently begun to attract attention is the growing proportion of the population that cannot get any insurance at a price that is affordable either to small employers or to themselves. By fracturing the insurance pool, the leading corporations have moved the nation closer to the precipice where the potential of private health insurance to cover most of the population is being questioned.[10]

Long-term Care. In the congressional debates about catastrophic benefits, the leading advocates emphasized that Medicare is grievously deficient when it comes to meeting the total health needs of the elderly due to its marginal contributions to nursing home, home, and congregate living care.

Admittedly, low-income and even moderate-income families can be bankrupted if a spouse requires, as in the case of Alzheimer's disease, three, four, or more years of institutionalization. But it is questionable whether the actual need is for health care services (there is no known treatment for Alzheimer's disease) or for personal services such as domestic help or periodic relief for a spouse or children who are the principal care givers.

Between 75 percent and 86 percent of all expenditures for the noninstitutionalized, enfeebled elderly is covered by the individuals themselves, their families, friends, and philanthropy. What proportion of these costs should be transferred to the federal budget, especially in the present situation of serious and continuing deficit, remains a moot question.

Rationing Expensive Care. The proposition is being advanced with increasing frequency (Aaron and Schwartz[11] and Callahan[12]) that given the astronomic costs of high-tech medicine, the United States must start to ration care. The usual proposal is for age-based rationing: to refuse people in their seventies or eighties such high-cost services as renal dialysis, open-heart surgery, and liver transplants.

However, the proponents of this view have adduced no evidence, much less conclusive evidence, that such a harsh approach is necessary or that it would be acceptable to the American public; that the continuing acceleration in health care costs is attributable to the investment of huge sums in treating people who are nearing the end of their lives; or that as the public becomes increasingly sophisticated about the unwarranted prolongation of life (consider the living will) it is reasonable to discriminate in the use of high-tech medicine among patients on the basis of their age. The fact is, our medicine—and the best of world medicine—is high-tech and will become even more so.

Prevention. Because of frustration over the steadily increasing costs of health care, with no proximate interruption of the trend in sight, many believers in prevention advocate that the society should provide monetary incentives (in the form of reduced insurance premiums) for those who pursue a healthy life-style. The matter, however, is not quite so simple. The Surgeon General has recently defined tobacco as an addictive substance, and Americans engage in many other habits and activities that are injurious to their health, from eating unwholesome foods to driving at excessive speeds. In theory there may be justification for differentiating in the expenditures for, and access to, health care among people with differing life-styles. Nevertheless, it is important to remember some obvious facts; many who jog develop orthopedic impairments; many who are overweight suffer from glandular, not eating, disturbances; a great number of chronic medical conditions are inherited; and even the most health-conscious, exercise-oriented, cautious individual is not immune to cancer or other devastating diseases.

The Canadian Health Care System. Aware that American health costs as a percentage of GNP are higher than those in any other advanced nation and that the ratio is likely to increase, a growing number of health analysts are looking with increasing favor on the Canadian health system, which, in their view, provides a level of care comparable to ours with access of the entire population at a cost of some three percentage points below the United States—circa 8 percent to 9 percent of the GNP.[13]

Several reservations must be noted. In terms of population

Canada is about the equivalent of the state of California—hardly a fair match with the United States, which contains another 49 states and 220 million people. Even there the system has its flaws. Emergency departments in major hospitals in major Canadian cities have had to be shut down for lack of beds, many of them filled with patients awaiting transfer to long-term care facilities that do not exist. Important teaching hospitals have been unable to purchase new equipment except as they have managed to cut back on their traditional services. There has been on-again, off-again confrontation between the medical profession and various provincial governments. True, universal access has been ensured, but the long-term outlook is not sanguine, at least not in the opinion of many of the medical profession's leaders.[14]

A Look Ahead

Despite all our efforts of recent years, then, health care costs continue to increase, with governmental estimates of $1 trillion for 1995 and $1.5 trillion for 2000, up from $0.5 trillion in 1987.[15] There is undoubtedly waste in the health care system, but no solid proposals have been advanced to recapture the $100 billion, plus or minus, that some believe can be saved.

I believe that we will not reshape our national health policy agenda unless and until we achieve a broad consensus on the key issues. Do the American people, for example, desire to ensure access to health care for the entire population? In that case they must agree to pick up a sizable additional tab, which they have thus far avoided. Concern for the nation's steadily increasing health care appears to be limited only to politicians and employers who must foot most of the bill. Public opinion polls, however, invariably state that the nation should spend more on health.

As long as the public places a higher value on ready access to physicians than on more subtle aspects of quality control, it is unlikely that state legislators will cut back on admissions to medical schools. And although many Americans would like to slow the rise in their health care costs, it is far from certain that to do so, large numbers would be willing to enroll in capitated plans that would restrict or deny them free choice of physicians or specialists.

It is not clear at what point on its steeply rising health-cost curve corporate America may seek to shift its participation in the financing of health care to government, federal and state, even while continuing to pay its share.

The problems connected with the financing of long-term care cannot be avoided much longer, but the solutions will not come easily given the potential costs, the embryonic stage of insurance coverage for long-term care, and the confusion between health and personal-care services. Likewise, there is little reason to believe that the American people will opt in favor of restricting access to expensive high-tech medicine on the basis of age; the issue, however, invites further discussion.

The growing enthusiasm for the Canadian approach (national health insurance with universal coverage) may be an important signal of growing public concern about the future direction of the U.S. health care system. However, it will require more profound destabilization of our health care system than we have experienced thus far before a political consensus on change emerges.

Notes · Index

Notes

1. The Destabilization of Health Care

Originally published in the *New England Journal of Medicine*, 315 (September 18, 1986): 757–761.

1. M. R. Schwarz, "Physician personnel and physician practice." In E. Ginzberg, ed., *From Physician Shortage to Patient Shortage: The Uncertain Future of Medical Practice* (Boulder, Colo.: Westview Press), pp. 35–74.
2. *Source Book of Health Insurance Data 1985–86* (Washington, D.C.: Health Insurance Association of America, 1985), p. 6.
3. *Report of the Task Force on Academic Health Centers: Prescription for Change* (New York: The Commonwealth Fund, 1985).
4. E. Ginzberg, "Is cost containment for real?" *JAMA*, 256 (1986): 254–255.
5. M. L. Millman, *Politics and the Expanding Physician Supply* (Totowa, N.J.: Allanheld, Osmun, 1980).
6. A. R. Tarlov, "HMO enrollment growth and physicians: The third compartment," *Health Affairs*, 5, no. 1 (1986): 23–35.
7. M. S. Feldstein, "A new approach to national health insurance," *Public Interest*, 23 (Spring 1971): 93–105.
8. A. C. Enthoven, "Consumer-choice health plan," *New England Journal of Medicine*, 298 (1978): 650–658, 709–720.
9. R. M. Gibson, K. R. Levit, H. Lazenby, and D. R. Waldo, "National health expenditures, 1983," *Health Care Financing Review*, 6, no. 2 (1984): 1–29.
10. C. Bradford, G. Caldwell, and J. Goldsmith, "The hospital capital crisis: Issues for trustees." *Harvard Business Review*, 60, no. 5 (1982): 56–68.
11. D. R. Cohodes and B. Kinkead, *Hospital Capital Formation in the 1980s* (Baltimore: Johns Hopkins University Press, 1984).
12. E. Ginzberg and Conservation of Human Resources Project Staff, *From*

Health Dollars to Health Services: New York City 1965–1985 (Totowa, N.J.: Rowman & Allanheld, 1986), pp. 54–62.

13. Institute of Medicine, *For-Profit Enterprise in Health Care* (Washington, D.C.: National Academy Press, 1986). B. H. Gray and W. J. McNerney, "For-profit enterprise in health care: The Institute of Medicine study," *New England Journal of Medicine* 314 (1986): 1523–1528.

14. United States General Accounting Office, *Hospital Merger Increased Medicare and Medicaid Payment for Capital Costs* (Washington, D.C.: General Accounting Office, 1983), publication no. GAO/HRD-84-10.

15. *Statistical Profile of the Investor-Owned Hospital Industry* (Washington, D.C.: Federation of American Hospitals, 1979–1980; 1981; 1982; 1983; 1984).

16. J. K. Iglehart, "Kaiser, HMOs and the public interest: A conversation with James A. Vohs," *Health Affairs*, 5, no. 1 (1986): 36–50.

17. U.S. Senate Committee on Finance, *The Social Security Act as Amended through January 4, 1975 and Related Laws* (Washington, D.C.: Government Printing Office, 1975).

18. D. A. Stockman, "Premises for a medical marketplace: A neoconservative's vision of how to transform the health system," *Health Affairs*, 1, no. 1 (1981): 5–18.

19. J. C. Goldsmith, "The changing role of the hospital." In E. Ginzberg, ed., *The U.S. Health Care System: A Look to the 1990s* (Totowa, NJ: Rowman & Allanheld, 1985), pp. 48–69.

20. J. B. Trauner, H. S. Luft, and S. Hunt, "A lifestyle decision: Facing the reality of physician oversupply in the San Francisco Bay Area." In E. Ginzberg, ed., *From Physician Shortage to Patient Shortage: The Uncertain Future of Medical Practice* (Boulder, Colo.: Westview Press, 1986), pp. 119–134.

21. S. C. Renn, C. J. Schramm, D. M. Watt, and R. Derzon, "The effects of ownership and system affiliation on the economic performance of hospitals," *Inquiry*, 22 (1985): 219–236.

22. See note 3, above.

23. E. Ginzberg, "Review of *Strained Mercy: The Economics of Canadian Health Care*," *New England Journal of Medicine*, 315 (1986): 715–716.

24. See note 3, above.

2. For-Profit Medicine

Originally published as "For-profit medicine: A reassessment" in the *New England Journal of Medicine*, 319 (September 22, 1988): 757–761.

1. R. Teitelman, "The SuperMeds," *Financial World*, June 10, 1986, pp. 22–29.

2. Annual report, *Nashville: Hospital Corporation of America*, 1985. Annual report, *Nashville: Hospital Corporation of America*, 1986. Annual report, *Louisville, Ky.: Humana*, 1985. Annual report, *Louisville, Ky.: Humana*, 1986. Annual report, *Los Angeles: National Medical Enterprises*, 1985. Annual report, *Los Angeles: National Medical Enterprises*,

1986. Annual report, *Beverly Hills, Calif.: American Medical International*, 1985. Annual report, *Beverly Hills, Calif.: American Medical International*, 1986.

3. A. Flexner, *Medical Education in the United States and Canada* (New York: Carnegie Foundation for the Advancement of Teaching, 1910, p. 173.

4. Health Care Financing Administration, Division of National Cost Estimates, "National health expenditures, 1986–2000," *Health Care Financing Review*, 8, no. 4 (1987): 1–36.

5. American Hospital Association, *Hospital Statistics: Data from the American Hospital Association 1986 Annual Survey* (Chicago: American Hospital Association, 1987).

6. See note 4, above.

7. See note 5, above.

8. See note 5, above.

9. General Accounting Office, *Hospital Merger Increased Medicare and Medicaid Payments for Capital Costs* (Washington, D.C.: General Accounting Office, 1983), publication no. GAO/HRD-84-10.

10. B. H. Gray, *For-Profit Enterprise in Health Care* (Washington, D.C.: National Academy Press, 1986), pp. 74–96.

11. E. Ginzberg and G. Vojta, *Beyond Human Scale: The Large Corporation at Risk* (New York: Basic Books, 1985).

12. See note 5, above.

13. See note 5, above.

14. H. S. Berliner, *Strategic Factors in U.S. Health Care: Human Resources, Capital and Technology* (Boulder, Colo.: Westview Press, 1987), p. 79.

15. H. S. Berliner and C. Regan, "Multinational operations of US for-profit hospital chains: Trends and implications," *American Journal of Public Health*, 77 (1987): 1280–1284.

16. H. S. Berliner and R. K. Burlage, "Proprietary hospital chains and academic medical centers," *International Journal of Health Services*, 17 (1987): 27–46.

17. See note 2, above.

18. A. S. Relman, "The new medical-industrial complex," *New England Journal of Medicine*, 303 (1980): 963–970. A. S. Relman, "Dealing with conflicts of interest," *New England Journal of Medicine*, 313 (1985): 749–751.

19. See note 4, above.

20. See note 4, above.

21. See note 4 above; see also *Source Book of Health Insurance Data, 1988 Update* (Washington, D.C.: Health Insurance Association of America, 1988).

3. American Medicine: The Power Shift

The Martin Memorial Lecture, originally published in the *Bulletin of the American College of Surgeons*, 70, no. 4 (April 1985).

1. J. Lister, "Private medical practice and the national health service," *New England Journal of Medicine*, 311 (1984): 1057–1061.

4. Privatization of Health Care

Originally published as "Privatization of Health Care: A U.S. Perspective" in *Annals of the New York Academy of Sciences*, 530 (June 15, 1988): 111–117.

1. E. Ginzberg, D. L. Hiestand, and B. G. Reubens, *The Pluralistic Economy* (New York: McGraw-Hill, 1965).
2. G. Rudney, "The scope and dimensions of non-profit activity. In W. W. Powell, ed., *The Nonprofit Sector: A Research Handbook* (New Haven: Yale University Press, 1987).
3. D. R. Waldo, K. R. Levit, and H. Lazenby, "National health expenditures, 1985," *Health Care Financing Review*, 8, no. 1 (1986): 1–21.
4. *U.S. Industrial Outlook 1987: Health and Medical Services* (Washington, D.C.: U.S. Department of Commerce).
5. *Statistical Abstract of the United States: 1987.* 107th ed. (Washington, D.C.: U.S. Bureau of the Census).
6. D. A. Stockman, "Premises for a medical marketplace: A neoconservative's vision of how to transform the health system, *Health Affairs*, 1, no. 1 (1981): 5–18.
7. E. Ginzberg, *American Medicine: The Power Shift* (Totowa, N.J.: Rowman & Allanheld, 1985).
8. See note 7, above.
9. R. M. Gibson, "National health expenditures, 1979," *Health Care Financing Review*, 2, no. 1 (1980): 1–36.
10. A. Enthoven, "Health tax policy mismatch," *Health Affairs*, 4, no. 4 (1985): 5–14.
11. *Source Book of Health Insurance Data, 1986–1987* (Washington, D.C.: Health Insurance Association of America).
12. *The Federal Register.* (Washington, D.C.: June 3, 1986).
13. *NIH Data Book 1986* (Washington, D.C.: U.S. Department of Health and Human Services. Public Health Service. National Institutes of Health).
14. A. E. Crowley, S. I. Etzel, and E. S. Petersen, "Undergraduate medical education," *Journal of the American Medical Association*, 246 (1981): 2913–2930. See also *Journal of the American Medical Association*, 254 (1985): 1565–1572.
15. E. Ginzberg, "A hard look at cost containment," *New England Journal of Medicine*, 316 (1987): 1151–1154.
16. E. Ginzberg, "Monetarization of medical care." In *American Medicine: The Power Shift* (Totowa, N.J.: Rowman & Allanheld, 1985).
17. K. Welling, "Recovery or remission? Short term outlook brightens for hospital management corp," *Barrons Weekly*, May 25, 1987.
18. *Humana 1985 Annual Report.* Louisville, KY: Humana, Inc.

19. S. E. Lind, "Fee-for-service research," *New England Journal of Medicine,* 314 (1986): 312–315.
20. R. K. Oldham, "Patient-funded cancer research," *New England Journal of Medicine,* 316 (1987): 46–47.
21. E. Ginzberg, "Competition: Policy or fantasy?" and, "The grand illusion of competition." In *American Medicine: The Power Shift* (Totowa, N.J.: Rowman & Allanheld, 1985). Ginzberg, E. Book review, *Strained Mercy: The Economics of Canadian Health Care,* by R. G. Evans, New England Journal of Medicine, 315 (1986): 715–716.

5. High-Tech Medicine

Initially prepared for a postponed symposium on technology and medicine.

6. Academic Health Centers: A Troubled Future

This chapter is composed of two articles originally published as: "Academic health centers: A troubled future," in *Health Affairs,* 4, no. 2 (Summer 1985): 5–21; and "Academic health centers—can they afford to relax?" *Journal of the American Medical Association,* 258, no. 14 (October 9, 1987): 1936–1937. Copyright 1987, American Medical Association.

1. J. W. Wilson, "Hospital chains struggle to stay in the pink," *Business Week,* 112 (January 14, 1985).
2. L. H. Aiken and K. D. Bays, "The medicare debate—round one," *New England Journal of Medicine,* 311 (1984): 1196–2000; and U.S. Congress, House, Committee on Ways and Means, Subcommittee on Health, *Proceedings of the Conference on the Future of Medicare* (Washington, D.C.: Government Printing Office, 1984).
3. J. C. Goldsmith, "Death of a paradigm: The challenge of competition," *Health Affairs,* (Fall 1984): 5–19.
4. A. Chandler, *The Visible Hand: The Managerial Revolution in American Business* (Cambridge: Harvard University Press, 1977).
5. E. Ginzberg, "Medical progress: How much money will it take?" *Journal of Medical Education* 59 (1984): 367–372.
6. R. Fein and G. Weber, *Financing of Medical Education: An Analysis of Alternate Policies* (New York: McGraw Hill, 1971).
7. A. Relman, "Who will pay for medical education in our teaching hospitals?" *Science,* 226 (1984): 220–223; and E. Ginzberg, "Graduate medical education in a period of constrained dollars," *Bulletin of the New York Academy of Medicine,* 59 (1983): 535–541.
8. A. G. Swanson, "Implications of the expanding physician supply for medical schools and medical students." In E. Ginzberg and M. Ostow,

eds., *The Coming Physician Surplus* (Totowa, N.J.: Rowman and Allanheld, 1984).

9. E. Ginzberg et al., *From Health Dollars to Health Services: New York City 1965–1985* (Totowa, N.J.: Rowman & Allanheld, in press).

10. "Annual report on medical education in the U.S.," *Journal of the American Medical Association* (1950–1975).

11. Association of American Medical Colleges, *Physicians for the Twenty-First Century* (Washington, D.C.: AAMC, 1984).

12. R. A. Stevens, "Defining and certifying the specialists." In *The Coming Physician Surplus* (see note 8, above).

13. M. Ostow, "Affiliation contracts." In E. Ginzberg et al., *Urban Health Services: The Case of New York* (New York: Columbia University Press, 1971).

14. E. Ginzberg and G. Vojta, *Beyond Human Scale: The Large Corporation at Risk* (New York: Basic Books, 1985).

15. Two recent joint ventures are Hoechst/Massachusetts General Hospital and Eugenics/Center for Biotechnology Research and Stanford University. For a discussion of the questions such agreements raise, see U.S. Department of Health and Human Services, Office of Technology Assessment, *Commercial Biotechnology* (Washington, D.C.: Government Printing Office, January 1984).

16. Graduate Medical Education National Advisory Committee (GMENAC), *Report of the Graduate Medical Education National Advisory Committee to the Secretary, Department of Health and Human Services* (Washington, D.C.: Government Printing Office, 1980).

17. For example, pathology increased its training period to five years and pediatrics requires a minimum of four residents per year for program accreditation.

18. E. Ginzberg, "The future supply of physicians: From pluralism to policy," *Health Affairs*, (Spring 1982): 6–19.

19. R. Heyssel, "Constrained resources in medical education and research," *Health Affairs*, (Winter 1984).

20. Ginzberg, "Medical progress: How much money will it take?"

21. Goldsmith, "Death of a Paradigm."

22. M. Rabkin, "Obstacles and opportunities for the teaching hospitals," *Hospitals*, (December 1, 1984): 86–88.

23. E. Ginzberg, "The high cost of dying," *Inquiry*, 17 (1980): 293–295.

24. Advisory Council on Social Security, *Medicare Benefits and Financing* (Washington, D.C.: 1983).

25. Heyssel, "Constrained resources."

26. W. B. Schwartz et al., *The Changing Geographic Distribution of Board-Certified Physicians* (Santa Monica, Calif.: Rand, 1980).

27. E. Ginzberg, "The monetarization of medical care," *New England Journal of Medicine*, 310 (1984): 1162–1165.

28. E. Ginzberg, "The decline of antiquity," *Social Studies*, 26 (1935): 82–90.

29. Ginzberg and Vojta, *Beyond Human Scale*.

30. Originally published in the *Journal of the American Medical Association*, 258, no. 14 (October 9, 1987): 1936–1937.
31. "Congress may block PPS rules: Reconciliation lags," *AHA News*, August 10, 1987, p. 1.
32. *Reducing the Deficit: Spending and Revenue Options.* Washington, D.C.: Congress of the United States; Congressional Budget Office, January 1987, pp. 63–69.

7. Foundations and the Nation's Health Agenda

Originally published in *Health Affairs*, Vol. 6, No. 4, Winter 1987, pp. 128–140.

1. B. L. Dooley, "Health giving patterns of philanthropic foundations," *Health Affairs*, 6 (Summer, 1987): 144–168.

8. The Community Health Care Center

Originally published as "The community health care center: current status and future directions" by Eli Ginzberg and Miriam Ostow, in *Journal of Health Politics, Policy and Law*, 10, no. 2 (Summer 1985): 283–298. Copyright 1985 by Duke University.

1. See E. M. Davis and M. L. Millman, *Health Care for the Urban Poor: Directions for Policy* (Totowa, N.J.: Rowman and Allanheld, 1983), for a larger overview of the MHSP.
2. See, for example, K. Davis and C. Schoen, *Health and the War on Poverty: A Ten Year Appraisal* (Washington, D.C.: Brookings Institution, 1978); D. Altman, "Health care for the poor," in S. Berki, ed., *Health Care Policy in America* (Beverly Hills: Sage Publications, 1983), pp. 103–121; and M. I. Roemer, *Ambulatory Health Services in America: Past, Present and Future* (Rockville, MD: Aspen Systems, 1981).
3. G. V. Fleming and R. M. Andersen, *The Municipal Health Services Program: Improving Access While Controlling Costs*, vols. 1 and 2 of the Final Report For the Health Care Financing Administration under HCFA 500-78-0097 and The Robert Wood Johnson Foundation RWJF #6798, April 1985.
4. Davis and Millman, *Health Care for the Urban Poor*, provides detail on the structure of the five programs.
5. E. Ginzberg, E. Davis, and M. Ostow, *Local Health Policy in Action: The Municipal Health Services Program* (Totowa, N.J.: Rowman and Allanheld, 1985).
6. The Robert Wood Johnson Foundation, "An assessment of the municipal health services program demonstration and its implications for local government," Final Report, October 1983.
7. E. Ginzberg and M. Ostow, eds., *The Coming Physician Surplus* (Totowa, N.J.: Rowman & Allanheld, 1984).

8. J. C. Goldsmith, *Can Hospitals Survive?* (Homewood, Ill.: Dow Jones-Irwin, 1981).

9. L. Etheredge, "Reagan, Congress and health spending," *Health Affairs*, 2 (Spring 1983): 14–24.

10. "Business-minded health care," *New York Times*, February 12, 1985, p. D1.

11. Ginzberg and Ostow, *The Coming Physician Surplus*.

12. See the discussion in L. E. Demkovich, "Hospitals that provide for the poor are reeling from uncompensated costs," *National Journal*, November 24, 1984, pp. 2245–2249.

13. L. D. Brown, "The managerial imperative and organizational innovation in health services," presented at the Cornell Conference on Health Policy, Cornell University Medical College, N.Y., March 7–8, 1985.

14. See, for example, J. Hadley and J. Feder, *Hospital Cost Shifting* (Washington, D.C.: Center for Health Policy Studies, Georgetown University, October 1984).

15. Goldsmith, *Can Hospitals Survive?*

16. S. Guttmacher, "No golden door: The health care and non-care of the undocumented," *Health/Pac Bulletin* 14 (March–April 1983): 15–24; see also Guttmacher, "Immigrant workers: health, law, and public policy," *Journal of Health Politics, Policy and Law*, 9 (Fall 1984): 503–514.

17. T. Martico, *The Medicare Fiscal Crisis and Approaches to Reform* (New York: Brookdale Institute on Aging and Adult Human Development, Columbia University, November 1984).

18. See J. W. Thomas et al., "Increasing medicare enrollment in HMOs: The need for capitation rates adjusted for health status," *Inquiry*, 20 (Fall 1983): 227–239.

19. J. K. Iglehart, "Medicaid in transition," *New England Journal of Medicine*, 309 (6 October 1983): 868–872.

20. For a more comprehensive analysis of efforts to help finance care for the indigent see G. Richards, "Indigent care legislation, 1984," *Hospitals*, October 16 1984, pp. 117–118.

21. A. Sager, "Forces shaping the reconfiguration of urban hospitals," *Health and the City, Urban Affairs Annual Review*, 25 (1983).

22. Ginzberg and Ostow, eds., *The Coming Physician Surplus*.

23. D. H. Talbot, "Hospitals," *Bulletin of the New York Academy of Medicine*, 61 (January–February, 1985): 23–30.

24. See, for example, L. Punch, "Hospitals may reduce indigent care as competition rules out cost shifting," *Modern Health Care*, November 1, 1984, p. 30.

25. Demkovitch, "Hospitals that provide for the poor," p. 2249.

26. See B. Vladeck and W. Carr, "Health," in C. Brecher and R. D. Horton, eds., *Setting Municipal Priorities, 1982* (New York: Russell Sage Foundation, 1981).

27. S. Mulstein, "The Uninsured and the financing of uncompensated care: Scope, costs and policy options," *Inquiry*, 21 (Fall, 1984): 214–229.

28. Popular opinion polls supporting national health insurance are cited in R. J. Blendon and D. E. Altman, "Public attitudes about health care costs," *New England Journal of Medicine*, 311 (August 30, 1984): 613–616.

9. Health Care in New York City

Originally published as "Health care in New York City: A system in flux," by Eli Ginzberg and Miriam Ostow, in *New York Affairs*, 9, no. 2 (1985): 58–73.

10. The Reform of Medical Education

Originally published as "The reform of medical education" by Robert H. Ebert and Eli Ginzberg in *Health Affairs*, supplement 1988, pp. 5–38.

1. The term "medical specialty" has two meanings, and it is important to distinguish between them. The major clinical specialties are internal medicine, surgery, obstetrics and gynecology, pediatrics, psychiatry, otolaryngology, and ophthalmology, but within each of these specialties there are subspecialties. For example, internal medicine is divided into such specialties as cardiology, gastroenterology, and endocrinology; surgery includes subspecialties of orthopedics, urology, cardiac surgery, plastic surgery, and so on. The surgical subspecialties of orthopedics and urology are so large and important that they are commonly given the status of separate academic departments, which are, in turn, divided into subspecialties.
2. Robert J. Blendon, "The changing role of private philanthropy in health affairs," *New England Journal of Medicine*, 292 (1975): 946–950.
3. August G. Swanson, "U.S. medical school applicants and matriculants, 1960–1985 and beyond," in Eli Ginzberg, ed., *From Physician Shortage to Patient Shortage* (Boulder, Colo.: Westview Press, 1986).
4. Alvin R. Tarlov, "HMO enrollment growth and physicians: The third compartment," *Health Affairs*, (Spring 1986): 23–35.
5. The Commonwealth Fund, *Report of the Task Force on Academic Health Centers: Prescription for Change* (New York: The Commonwealth Fund, 1985).

11. The Politics of Physician Supply

A paper prepared for the International Conference on "The Political Dynamics of Physician Manpower Policy," London, England, May 24–27, 1988. Organizing Committee: Marilynn Rosenthal, Irene Butter, Mark Field, Bui Dang Ha Doan, Jan Grund, M.D. Shortened version in press.

Dr. James Sammons, the Executive Vice President of the American Medical Association and Dr. James F. Rodgers, Director of the Center for Health Policy Research, greatly facilitated my securing access to key policy documents involving the AMA's changing positions on the issue of physician supply.

1. M. Fishbein, *A History of the American Medical Association* (Philadelphia: W. B. Saunders, 1947).
2. A. Flexner, *Medical Education in the United States and Canada* (Flexner Report) (New York, N.Y.: The Carnegie Foundation for the Advancement of Teaching, 1910), p. x.
3. V. Johnson, The Council on Medical Education and Hospitals. In M. Fishbein, *A History of the American Medical Association*, p. 899.
4. Ibid., p. 901.
5. *Medical Education: Final Report of the Commission on Medical Education* (New York: N.Y.: Office of the Director of the Study, 1932), p. 1.
6. Ibid., pp. 64, 93, 100, 119, 120.
7. M. Fishbein, *A History of the American Medical Association.*
8. E. Rayack, *Professional Power and American Medicine: The Economics of the American Medical Association* (Cleveland: World Publishing Company, 1967).
9. J. H. Morton, "Politics and medical manpower," *Federal Bulletin* 73 (1986): 137–140.
10. O. W. Ewing, *The Nation's Health: A Ten-Year Program* (Ewing Report) (Washington, D.C.: Federal Security Agency, 1948).
11. U. S. President's Commission on the Health Needs of the Nation, *Building America's Health: A Report to the President* (Magnuson Report), 5 vols. (Washington, D.C.: U.S. Government Printing Office, 1952–53).
12. F. G. Dickinson, *An Analysis of the Ewing Report* (Chicago: American Medical Association, bulletin 69, 1949).
13. *The Advancement of Medical Education and Research through the Department of Health, Education and Welfare* (Bayne-Jones Report), final report of the secretary's consultants on medical research and education (Washington, D.C.: U.S. Government Printing Office, June 1958).
14. U.S. Department of Health, Education and Welfare, *Physicians for a Growing America* (Bane Report), report of the Surgeon General's consultant group on medical education (Washington, D.C.: U.S. Government Printing Office, 1959).
15. *Federal Support of Medical Research* (Jones Report), report of the Committee on Appropriations, Subcommittee on Department of Health, Education and Welfare (Washington, D.C.: U.S. Government Printing Office, 1960).
16. *A National Program to Conquer Heart Disease, Cancer and Stroke,* report of the President's Commission on Heart Disease, Cancer and

Stroke. *Report of the Subcommittee on Manpower* (Washington, D.C.: U.S. Government Printing Office, 1965).

17. L. T. Coggeshall, *Planning for Medical Progress through Education* (Evanston, Ill.: Association of American Medical Colleges, 1965).

18. *Report of the National Advisory Commission on Health Manpower* (Washington, D.C.: U.S. Government Printing Office, November 1967).

19. *Higher Education and the Nation's Health: Policies for Medical and Dental Education*, a special report and recommendations by the Carnegie Commission on Higher Education (New York, N.Y.: McGraw-Hill, 1970).

20. *Costs of Education in the Health Professions*, a report by the Institute of Medicine, U.S. Department of Health, Education, and Welfare. (Washington, D.C.: DHEW Publication no. (HRA) 74-32, January 1974).

21. F. J. L. Blasingame, "Physicians and the marketplace," *Journal of the American Medical Association* 204 (1968): 143–146.

22. B. Senior and B. A. Smith, "The number of physicians as a constraint on delivery of health care: How many physicians are enough?" *Journal of the American Medical Association* 222 (1972): 178–183.

23. E. Ginzberg, "A cautionary view of medical care," *New England Journal of Medicine* 262 (1960): 367–368.

24. E. Ginzberg, "Physician shortage reconsidered," *New England Journal of Medicine* 275 (1966): 85–87.

25. M. L. Millman, *Politics and the Expanding Physician Supply* (Montclair, N.J.: Allanheld Osmun, 1980).

26. *GMENAC Summary Report*, report of the Graduate Medical Education National Advisory Committee to the Secretary, Department of Health and Human Services (Washington, D.C.: U.S. Government Printing Office, September 1980).

27. G. D. Lundberg, "GMENAC, AMA Policy, and the Pitfalls of Parkinsonism," *Journal of the American Medical Association* 250 (1983): 2633–2634.

28. E. Ginzberg, "A new physician supply policy is needed," *Journal of the American Medical Association* 250 (1983): 2621–2622.

12. Nursing

Originally published as "Nurses for the future—facing the facts and figures," *Supplement of American Journal of Nursing*, December 1987, pp. 1596–1600.

13. Clinical Decision Making in Catastrophic Situations

Originally submitted on behalf of a six-person Policy Group, Eli Ginzberg, Chair, at a conference convened by the American Geriatrics Society, April 17–18, 1987. The Report of the Conference, "Clinical decision-making in catastrophic situations; the relevance of age," by

Jeremiah A. Barondess, M. D., Paul Kalb, M. D., William B. Weil, M.D., Christine Cassel, M.D., and Eli Ginzberg, Ph.D., was published in the *Journal of the American Geriatric Society*, 36, no. 10 (1988).

14. Rationing Cancer Care

Originally published as Chapter 9 in *Cost vs. Benefit in Cancer Care*, ed. Dr. Basil Stoll (London: MacMillan, 1988).

1. National Center for Health Statistics, "National medical care and expenditure survey, 1980. In *Costs of Illness, United States, 1980*, DHHS Pub. no. 86-20403 (Washington, D.C.: Office of Health Research, Statistics and Technology, 1986).
2. D. M. Eddy, "Screening for cancer in adults." In Ciba Foundation Symposium 110, *The Value of Preventive Medicine* (London: Pitman, 1985).
3. American Cancer Society, *1986 Cancer Facts & Figures* (New York: American Cancer Society, 1986).
4. B. A. Stoll, *Screening and Monitoring of Cancer* (New York: John Wiley, 1985), pp. 135–152.
5. Stuart E. Lind, "Fee-for-service research," *New England Journal of Medicine* 314 (1986): 312.

15. Health Care for the Elderly

Originally published as Chapter 25 in *Caring for the Elderly: Reshaping Health Policy*, ed. Carl Eisendorfer, David Kessler, and Abby Spector (Baltimore: The Johns Hopkins Press, 1989).

1. United States Department of Commerce, *Statistical Abstract of the United States, 1987* (Washington, D.C.: Government Printing Office, 1987), p. 446.
2. Ibid.
3. Ibid.
4. Ibid., pp 94, 99.
5. United States General Accounting Office, *The Elderly Should Benefit from Expanded Home Health Care but Increasing These Services Will Not Insure Cost Reductions*, report to the Chairman of the Committee on Labor and Human Resources, United States Senate (Washington, D.C.: GAO/IPE-83-1), pp. 26–31.
6. *Statistical Abstract*, p. 99 (see note 1, above).
7. J. Lubitz and R. Prihoda, "The use and costs of medicare services in the last 2 years of life," *Health Care Financing Review*, 5, no. 3 (1984): 117–131.
8. D. Waldo, and H. C. Lazenby, "Demographic characteristics and health care use expenditures by the aged in the United States: 1977–1984," *Health Care Financing Review*, 6, no. 1 (1984): 1–34.
9. J. W. Thomas, R. Lichtenstein, L. Wyszewianski, and S. E. Berki, "In-

creasing medicare enrollment in HMOs: The need for capitation rates adjusted for health status, *Inquiry,* 20 (Fall 1983): 227–239.

16. Psychiatry before the Year 2000

Originally published as "Psychiatry before the year 2000: The long view" in *Hospital and Community Psychiatry,* 38, no. 7 (July 1987); 725–728.

1. E. Ginzberg, *Understanding Human Resources* (Lanham, Md.: ABT Books, 1985).
2. E. Ginzberg, *Health Manpower and Health Policy* (Montclair, N.J.: Allanheld Osmun, 1978).
3. See note 2, above.
4. See note 2, above.
5. H. A. Foley and S. S. Sharfstein, *Madness and Government* (Washington, D.C.: American Psychiatric Press, 1983).
6. E. Ginzberg, T. J. Noyelle, and T. M. Stanback, Jr., *Technology and Employment* (Boulder, Colo.: Westview, 1986).
7. C. A. Taube and S. A. Barrett, *Mental Health, United States, 1983,* DHHS Publication ADM 83-1275 (Washington, D.C.: U.S. Government Printing Office, 1983). C. A. Taube, L. Kessler and M. Feuerberg. *Utilization and Expenditures for Ambulatory Mental Health Care During 1980,* National Medical Care Utilization and Expenditure Survey, Data Report 5, DHHS Publication PHS 84-20000 (Washington, D.C.: U.S. Government Printing Office, June 1984).
8. W. R. Curtis, "The deinstitutionalization story," *Public Interest* 85 (1986): 34–49.
9. L. R. Marcos and N. L. Cohen, "Taking the suspected mentally ill off the streets to public general hospitals," *New England Journal of Medicine* 315 (1986): 1158–1161.
10. *Prescription for Change: Report of the Task Force on Academic Health Centers* (New York: The Commonwealth Fund, 1985).

17. Medical Care for the Poor

Originally published under the title "Medical care for the poor: No magic bullets" in the *Journal of the American Medical Association,* 259, no. 22 (June 10, 1988): 3309–3311. Copyright 1988, American Medical Association.

18. Balancing Dollars and Quality

Prepared for cancelled conference on "Management of health care services without denying quality," June 1988, Mid-West Bio-Ethics Center, Kansas City.

19. A Hard Look at Cost Containment

Originally published in the *New England Journal of Medicine*, 316 (April 30, 1987): 1151–1154.

1. D. A. Stockman, "Premises for a medical marketplace: A neoconservative's vision of how to transform the health system," *Health Affairs*, (Millwood) 1, no. 1 (1981): 5–18; E. Ginzberg, "Letters: Stockman's medical marketplace reexamined," *Health Affairs*, (Millwood) 1, no. 2 (1982): 118–120.
2. E. Ginzberg, "Cost containment—imaginary and real," *New England Journal of Medicine*, 308: (1983) 1220–1224.
3. American Hospital Association, *Hospital Statistics* (Chicago: American Hospital Association, 1986).
4. W. B. Schwartz, "The inevitable failure of current cost-containment strategies," *JAMA* 257 (1987): 220–224.
5. "Economics," *Hospitals*, February 5, 1987, p. 36.
6. See note 5, above.
7. A. C. Enthoven, *Health Plan: The Only Practical Solution to the Soaring Cost of Health Care* (Reading, Mass.: Addison-Wesley, 1980).
8. H. S. Luft, "Trends in medical care costs: do HMOs lower rate of growth?" *Medical Care*, 18 (1980): 1–16. J. P. Newhouse, W. B. Schwartz, A. P. Williams, and C. Witsberger, "Are fee-for-service costs increasing faster than HMO costs?" *Medical Care*, 23 (1985): 960–966.
9. Center for Health Services Research and Development, ed. S. G. Vahovich, *Profile of Medical Practice* (Chicago: American Medical Association, 1973). Center for Health Policy Research, ed. M. L. Gonzalez, and D. W. Emmons, *Socioeconomic characteristics of medical practice* (Chicago: American Medical Association, 1986).
10. H. S. Luft and P. Arno, "Impact of increasing physician supply," *Health Affairs* (Millwood), 5, no. 4 (1986): 31–46.
11. J. K. Iglehart, "Kaiser, HMOs, and the public interest: A conversation with James A. Vohs," *Health Affairs* (Millwood) 5, no. 1 (1986): 44.
12. S. C. Renn, C. J. Schramm, D. M. Watt, and R. Derzon, "The effects of ownership and system affiliation on the economic performance of hospitals," *Inquiry*, 22 (1985): 219–236.
13. R. E. Herzlinger and W. S. Krasker, "Who profits from nonprofits?" *Harvard Business Review*, January–February 1987, pp. 93–105.
14. R. J. Blendon, "Policy choices for the 1990s: an uncertain look into America's future." In E. Ginzberg, *The U.S. Health Care System: A Look to the 1990s* (Totowa, N.J.: Rowman and Allanheld, 1985).

20. U. S. Health Policy: Expectations and Realities

Originally published in the *Journal of American Medical Asociation* 260 (December 23–30, 1988): 3647–3650. Copyright 1988, American Medical Associations.

1. Bureau of Health Professions, Health Resources and Services Administration, U.S. Department of Health and Human Services, unpublished data, 1988; Bureau of the Census, U.S. Department of Commerce, unpublished data, 1988.
2. Division of National Cost Estimates, Office of the Actuary, Health Care Financing Administration, "National health expenditures, 1986–2000," *Health Care Financing Review*, 8, no. 4 (1987): 1–29.
3. See note 2, above.
4. J. A. Califano, *America's Health Care Revolution: Who Lives? Who Dies? Who Pays?* (New York: Random House, 1986).
5. M. Chassin, R. H. Brook, R. E. Park, et al. "Variations in the use of medical and surgical services by the medicare population," *New England Journal of Medicine*, 314 (1986): 285–290.
6. J. E. Wennberg, "Dealing with medical practice variations: A proposal for action," *Health Affairs*, 3, no. 2 (1984): 6–32.
7. W. B. Schwartz, F. A. Sloan, and D. N. Mendelson, "Why there will be little or no physician shortage between now and the year 2000," *New England Journal of Medicine* 318 (1988): 892–897. E. P. Schloss, "Beyond GMENAC—another physician shortage from 2010 to 2030?" *New England Journal of Medicine* 318 (1988) 920–992.
8. L. R. Gruber, M. Shadle, and C. L. Polich, "From movement to industry: The growth of HMOs," *Health Affairs*, 7, no. 3 (1988): 197–208.
9. A. C. Enthoven, *Health Plan: The Only Practical Solution to the Soaring Cost of Medical Care* (Reading, Mass.: Addison-Wesley, 1980).
10. R. Fein, *Medical Care, Medical Costs: The Search for a Health Insurance Policy* (Cambridge: Harvard University Press, 1987).
11. H. J. Aaron and W. B. Schwartz. *The Painful Prescription: Rationing Hospital Care.* (Brookings Institution, Washington, D.C., 1984).
12. D. Callahan, *Setting Limits: Medical Goals in an Aging Society* (New York: Simon & Schuster, 1987).
13. G. J. Schieber and J-P. Poullier, "Trends in international health care spending," *Health Affairs*, 6, no. 3 (1987): 105–112.
14. *Health Care Reform: The Challenge for North America*, report of a Canada–United States Conference, November 18–19, 1987 (New York: Americas Society/Canadian Affairs, 1987).
15. Division of National Cost Estimates, Office of the Actuary, Health Care Financing Administration, "National health expenditures, 1986–2000," *Health Care Financing Review*, 8, no. 4 (1987): 1–29.

Index

Heterick Memorial Library
Ohio Northern University

DUE	RETURNED	DUE	RETURNED
1.		13.	
2.		14.	
3.		15.	
4.		16.	
5.		17.	
6.		18.	
7.		19.	
8.		20.	
9.		21.	
10.		22.	
		23.	
		24.	